W9-AOO-322

Uwe Streitferdt

Healthy Dog, Happy Dog

A Complete Guide to Dog Diseases and Their Treatment

Contributing authors:
Christine Metzger
Claus-Michael Pautzke
Drawings by Gyorgy Jankovics
and color photos by renowned
animal photographers

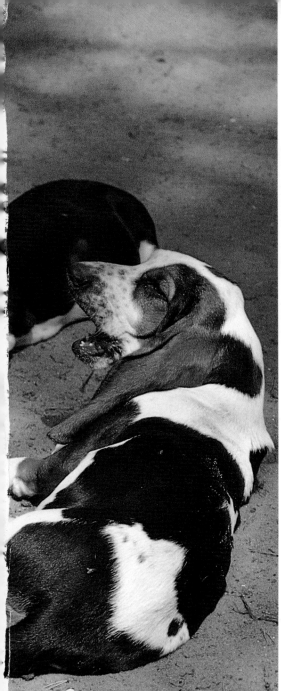

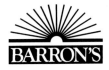

BARRON'S

Preface and Contents

What should you do if your dog suddenly starts behaving differently or if every step causes it obvious pain? This book tells you how you can help your dog when it gets sick.

The section devoted to practical advice contains useful general information:

How to feed your dog properly, plans for different diets, important tips on how to care for a healthy as well as a sick dog, and first-aid steps that help you to deal with an emergency. Also a table of symptoms will help you to recognize diseases quickly and to respond to them promptly.

The section on diseases describes the most important dog diseases and offers detailed summaries of possible treatments, and indicates when a veterinarian should be consulted. Technical terms often used by veterinarians are explained in a glossary.

Note: This book offers a conventional veterinary approach to the treatment of canine diseases, and then provides complementary homeopathic advice that broadens the range of effective care. However, homeopathy should be considered an adjunct to veterinary treatment and not an alternative to it. When in doubt, or if there is no response to home treatment, consult your veterinarian.

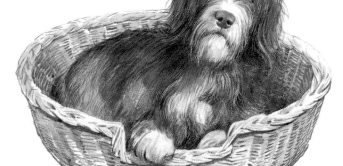

Guide to the Section on Diseases

Quick Recognition of Diseases

Symptom	Possible Causes That You Can Correct Yourself	Cause for Alarm If These Symptoms Also Are Present
Dog refuses food	Dog has had enough to eat or is spoiled and fussy; new kind of food; food too hot	Fever; vomiting; apathy Increased thirst; vomiting; no stool
Dog eats voraciously	Dog has not been fed for some time; is gluttonous by nature; is neutered	Dog drinks a lot, is obese, has a potbelly, is losing hair
Does not drink	Sufficient moisture in the food	Salivating; trouble swallowing; coughs; chokes
Drinks a lot	Overheating after playing hard; dog has eaten a lot of dry food	Vomiting and below-normal temperature Apathy; staggering; below-normal temperature In females: vomiting; fever; apathy
Diarrhea	Too much milk; cold food; eating snow; sudden change in diet; stress	Blood in stool; vomiting; dehydration; anemia
Vomiting	Eating grass; eating too fast	Yellowish white or bloody mucus in the vomit Apathy; diarrhea; high fever Refusal to eat; no stool; taut belly
Coughing	Choking, especially when drinking water fast	Dry cough and chocking up mucus Fits of dry coughing and choking up bloody mucus Mucopurulent inflammation of conjunctiva and nasal passages; labored breathing; fever Deep, wet cough; labored breathing
Foul smell from the mouth	Eating feces, carrion, or other foul-smelling things	Drooling, possibly with blood in saliva Vomiting; excessive drinking; putrid or urine-like smell from the mouth

Possible Diagnosis and Treatment	Description of Disease
Serious general infection. Call the veterinarian.	Pages 98, 99
Serious kidney or liver disease, pyometra (accumulation of pus in the uterus). Call the veterinarian.	Pages 66, 50, 72
Foreign body in the digestive tract. Call the veterinarian.	Page 46
Suspect hormonal disorder (thyroid deficiency, hyperfunction of the adrenal cortex). Call the veterinarian.	Pages 85, 86
Foreign body in the throat, paralysis of the esophagus (rabies). Call the veterinarian.	Pages 42, 43, 99
Kidney disease (with uremia): Call the veterinarian.	Page 66
Diabetes. Call the veterinarian.	Page 87
Pyometra. Call the veterinarian.	Page 72
Worms; infection of gastrointestinal tract; disease of the liver or pancreas; poisoning. Call the veterinarian.	Pages 101, 102, 44, 46, 47, 50, 51, 30, 31
Gastritis; foreign body in the stomach; liver or kidney disease; poisoning. Call the veterinarian	Pages 44, 43, 50, 51, 30, 31
Serious virus infection. Call the veterinarian.	Pages 98, 99
Foreign body in intestine. Call the veterinarian.	Page 46
Inflammation of the throat; tonsillitis or laryngitis (kennel cough). Call the veterinarian.	Pages 53, 100
Foreign body or tumor in the throat. Call the veterinarian.	Pages 42, 43
A cold; bronchitis; or pneumonia (possibly distemper). Call the veterinarian.	Pages 55, 56, 98
Heart disease and fluid in the lungs. Call the veterinarian.	Pages 58–59, 56
Tartar on teeth; periodontosis; infected tooth; foreign body or tumor in oral cavity. Call the veterinarian.	Pages 40, 41, 42, 43
Gastritis; kidney disease/uremia. Call the veterinarian.	Pages 44, 66

Symptom	Possible Causes That You Can Correct Yourself	Cause for Alarm If These Symptoms Also Are Present
Bloating	Feeding too much meat or carbohydrates; sudden change in diet	Diarrhea and light, pasty stool Especially in large dogs: choking up mucus; distended abdomen; apathy; breathing with moaning sound. Emergency! Call the vet!
Straining with no stool or urine	Constipation because of lack of exercise; dry food and not enough drinking; labor pains	Discharge of bloody slime or blood from the anus Bloody or dribbling urine
Large quantity of urine	Dog has drunk a lot, as in hot weather or after playing hard	Small frequent urination, perhaps bloody Large amounts of urine; increased thirst; apathy; poor appetite In females: Large amounts of urine and bloody or purulent discharge from the vagina
Labored breathing	Panting caused by over-heating, overexertion, or excitement	Fever; coughing; sneezing; choking Deep, wet cough; racing pulse Pumping breathing/abdomen sucking in Pale mucous membranes, racing pulse
Noisy breathing/ sneezing	Dog has sniffed or inhaled a foreign body	Mucopurulent and bloody discharge from nose; repeated noisy exhaling through nose Difficulties only in one nostril
Weakness of the back legs	Exhaustion after playing hard or dog is old and frail	Bent, tense, and aching back Difficulty getting up after lying down for some time Staggering, muscle spasms, tendency to cramps
Reeling/ staggering	Normal after getting up and when shaking the head	Walking in circles; standing apathetically in a corner; tendency to epileptic fits
Itching	Scratching ears because they are dirty; ticks or foreign objects; minor surface wounds	Itching all over; biting the fur Redness and areas of eczema on abdomen Places scratched raw especially on head and neck
Biting paws	Nails too long, matted hair and foreign objects between pads	Wetness and abscesses between toes Places with thickened, constantly raw skin on the foot joints

Possible Diagnosis and Treatment	**Description of Disease**
Chronic pancreatitis or liver disease	Pages 51, 50
Gastric torsion. Call the veterinarian.	Page 45
Constipation because of bones in stool. Call the veterinarian.	Page 48
Stones in bladder or urethra. Call the veterinarian.	Pages 64–65
Bladder infection, perhaps with bladder stones. Call the veterinarian.	Page 64
Chronic kidney or liver disease, hormonal problems (hyperfunction of adrenal cortex, diabetes). Call the veterinarian.	Pages 66, 50, 86, 87
Pyometra. Call the veterinarian.	Page 72
Cold, infection of airways (kennel cough). Call the veterinarian.	Pages 52–55, 100
Heart disease, fluid in the lungs. Call the veterinarian.	Pages 58, 56
Tear in lungs or diaphragm after an accident. Call the veterinarian.	Page 58
Internal bleeding after an accident or poisoning. Call the veterinarian.	Pages 27, 30, 31
Rhinitis	Page 52
Tumor or foreign body in the nose. Call the veterinarian.	Page 52
Herniated disc. Call the veterinarian.	Page 94
Chronic arthritis in hip or the knee joints.	Pages 92, 93
Chronic heart disease or meningitis (e.g., distemper). Call the veterinarian.	Pages 58–59, 95, 98
Concussion; meningitis; insufficient blood flow to the brain (arteriosclerosis, heart disease). Call the veterinarian.	Pages 28, 95, 98, 60, 58–59
Infestation with fleas or lice.	Pages 81, 82
Skin allergy caused by direct contact with irritant.	Page 83
Indirect contact allergy or autoimmune reaction of the skin.	Pages 83, 84
Foreign body (i.e., thorn) in paw.	Page 80
Inflamed skin caused by psychological problems (biting).	Page 80

A Healthy Dog

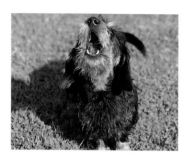

J ust look at him! Isn't he a fine fellow? His eyes are clear and bright, his coat shines, and his teeth are sparkling white. And he's already seven years old. His owners ascribe his good health to his varied and well-balanced diet. But that's not all there is to it. He has a good life—every day he's taken for a long walk and he gets brushed and groomed. Once a year he's taken to the veterinarian, even if there's nothing wrong with him. That's because his owners want him to stay healthy for a long time.

Behavior and Appearance

A healthy dog is a cheerful dog. It watches what goes on around it with alert eyes and greets family members with a wagging tail when they return home. When the mistress or master indicates that it's time for a walk, the dog leaps up eagerly. A healthy dog moves with ease, likes to play, and eats with a hearty appetite.

A glossy coat and clear eyes are signs of health in a dog. The bodily orifices—mouth, nose, eyes, ears, and anus, penis, or vagina—are clean and with no trace of wet or crusty discharge or of pus. Turn to page 11 to find out what your dog's appearance can tell you about its state of health.

Well-being—the Role of Affection and Training

Physical and emotional well-being are closely linked in all creatures. Dogs were originally pack animals that lived together in close-knit social groups, and our domestic dogs still need the approval and love of "their" humans to be emotionally well-adjusted. Dogs want to be petted and praised and are always happiest when they can be close to their owner.

Any grooming you do adds to your dog's well-being. If you brush its coat or clean its eyes and ears, your dog interprets this as acts of love, too. To find out more about grooming, turn to pages 18 and 19.

Another form of affection a dog benefits from is consistent and loving training, training that is based not on punishment but on praise. If you get your dog as a puppy, start teaching it early. You can begin housebreaking a puppy by the time it's eight weeks old, and at three months old, it should learn the commands "Sit," "Stay," and "Come." A companion dog also has to be able to stay by itself without barking and to walk on a leash without pulling.

Where the Dog Lives

If a dog is kept outside it will need a doghouse for protection and comfort. The doghouse should be big enough and well insulated against dampness, heat, and cold. The inside has to be clean, dry, and free from vermin.

A dog that has no doghouse to which it can retreat needs some kind of bed indoors. This can be a basket, a box, or a blanket, which must be placed somewhere that feels safe to the dog. Dogs like to lie under a bench or in a corner. The sleeping place should not be too warm or too cold, and should be free of drafts, which are bad for a dog's health. The

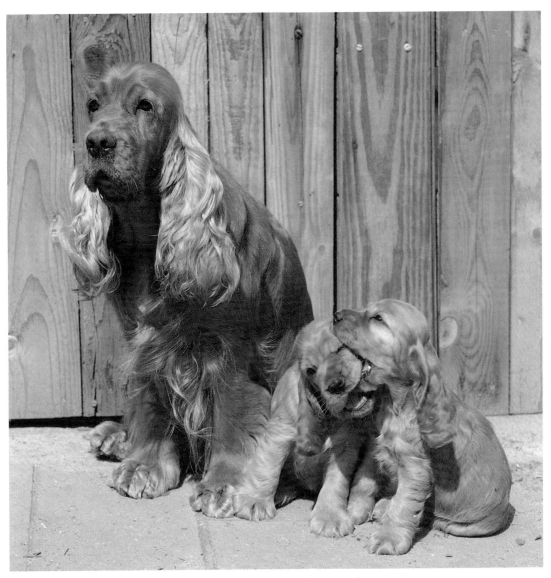

A proud mother with her playfully scuffling puppies. At this age play is the most important part of life.

bed also has to be big enough for the animal to stretch out full length. If there are several places that the dog can choose to lie on, this is ideal.

Closeness to people is very important to dogs. If a dog is alone much of the day, it should be allowed to sleep in a corner of the bedroom at night. Whether or not to allow the dog onto your bed is up to you. There is no health reason against a dog sleeping on the bed as long as the animal is well groomed, properly vaccinated and dewormed, and free from fleas, ticks, and lice.

Daily Walks

To stay healthy and fit, a dog has to get regular and sufficient exercise. Regular means at least one long walk a day. You can't skip the walk even if you have a yard where the dog can be outside. The length of the walk depends on the dog's breed, size, and age. Hunting and racing dogs need outings of up to two hours to work off their excess energy. Smaller and old dogs like shorter walks. When you take your dog out, it should always be able to run part of the way off the leash and to race across fields and through woods and bushes without restraint, if you live in the country. But in the city, because of cars and

trucks—and even other dogs that may carry transmissible diseases or harm your pet, dogs need to be walked on a leash.

In addition to the long walk, a dog has to be let out of the house at least four times a day to relieve itself.

Playing with the Dog

A healthy, lively dog wants to be kept busy and stimulated, and it will try to initiate play. Whether you throw a ball or stick on your daily walk, play tug of war with a rag, or hide a bone for the dog to find, you'll always find your dog an eager playmate. But you have to give some thought to the choice of toys. Toys should not be too small or the dog might swallow them. Objects with sharp edges are also to be avoided. Needless to say, toys should not contain toxic substances. In addition to toys for playing with you, the dog should get something to chew on, such as a rawhide "bone," to work on by itself. A good chew toy helps keep the teeth clean and helps prevents the buildup of tartar (page 40).

Dogs and Children

Dogs and children are ideal playmates. Anyone who has grown up with a dog knows that nothing else can match

such a friendship. As long as the dog is healthy and regularly vaccinated and dewormed, there is no reason to worry about letting children grow up with dogs.

An ideal dog for children has to combine a number of qualities. It should be an untiring playmate, never become aggressive, and not be noise sensitive or nervous. As a general rule, herding dogs, like collies and sheep dogs and their crosses, are especially good with children. But ultimately how a dog behaves with children depends on the temperament of the individual animal.

Another important factor is how the adults treat the children and the dog. If there is a new baby in the house, for example, it is important not to neglect the dog so no jealousy will arise. The dog has to learn to respect the child. But it's just as important to make clear to the child—as soon as he or she is old enough to understand— that a dog is a living being with feelings that also have to be respected. A dog must never be regarded as a toy.

Full responsibility for looking after a dog should not be given to a child unless he or she is capable and mature.

Is Your Dog Healthy?

*G*o through this test conscientiously, and make it a habit later on to watch your dog with these criteria in mind whenever you groom it or play with it. It will help you notice promptly any deviation from the dog's normal appearance or behavior.

Part 1

a) The coat should be glossy and hug the body in an even, dense layer. Is your dog's coat dull looking and ragged?

☐ Yes ☐ No

b) Offer your dog a treat that it usually takes eagerly. Is your dog refusing to eat it?

☐ Yes ☐ No

c) Suggest going for a walk in your usual way. Is the dog failing to respond and just lying down apathetically?

☐ Yes ☐ No

Part 2

a) Pull the lower eyelid down gently. Do the eyes look dull and are the conjunctiva red or yellow?

☐ Yes ☐ No

b) Is the area around the anus dirty or sticky?

☐ Yes ☐ No

c) Tell your dog to climb up the stairs or jump into the car. Is it refusing to do so even though it has ridden in a car and climbed stairs before?

☐ Yes ☐ No

Part 3

a) Are the dog's eyes, nostrils, or ears sticky with discharge or pus?

☐ Yes ☐ No

b) Is the skin red, scratched sore, purulent, or scabby?

☐ Yes ☐ No

c) Are the gums red and sore, does the dog drool, and is there a foul odor from its mouth?

☐ Yes ☐ No

d) Is the dog vomiting? Does it sometimes have diarrhea and bloating with rumbling intestinal sounds?

☐ Yes ☐ No

e) Does the dog pant even if it hasn't been racing around, or does it breathe heavily even after minor exertion?

☐ Yes ☐ No

f) Does your dog limp sometimes or does it have difficulties getting up and lying down?

☐ Yes ☐ No

g) Is your dog's temperature below 100.4°F (38°C) or above 102.2°F (39°C)? (See page 106 for taking the temperature.)

☐ Yes ☐ No

Evaluation of the Test

Your Dog Is Healthy
If you have answered all the questions with "No's," you can assume that your dog is healthy.

Reason for Concern
If you have marked "Yes" only in Part 1, there is no immediate cause for concern. The dog may just be having a "bad day." Repeat the test on the next three days. If the "Yes's" persist, take your dog to the veterinarian, especially if some symptoms of Part 2 or 3 turn up.

If you have marked one or more "Yes's" in Part 2, you should plan on a visit to the veterinarian soon. Only the veterinarian can tell if there is something seriously wrong.

Act Quickly
If you have even one "Yes" in Part 3, don't ignore it. Your dog is not well, and the change or changes you have noticed may indicate a serious illness. Call the veterinarian immediately, and also consult the table of symptoms on pages 4 to 7.

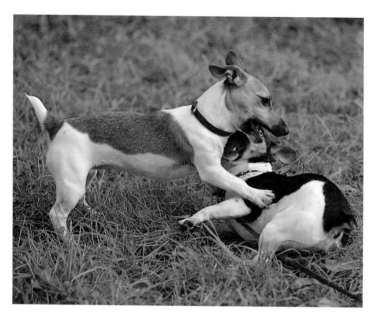

When playing and fighting, dogs exercise all the muscles in their bodies without even being aware of it.

The Proper Diet

We are what we eat. This is true of animals as well as of people. For a dog to grow properly, feel well, and stay healthy, it is extremely important that it be fed correctly, that is, in accordance with its natural needs.

The Right Food for Dogs

Dogs are carnivores, but they should not eat only muscle meat. A dog's digestive system resembles that of its ancestor, the wolf, and is adapted to digesting small plant-eating animals. These small prey animals are eaten whole—skin, fur, tendons, bones, and all. The contents of the prey's stomach and intestines are still largely undigested and consist primarily of plant matter. By eating the entire animal, wolves get roughage, proteins, carbohydrates, fats, minerals like calcium and phosphorus, vitamins, and trace elements.

Commercial Dog Food or Home-cooked Meals?

Commercial dog food has many advantages. It is convenient, doesn't take any time to prepare, and contains everything a dog needs. It is sold as wet food in cans, in the form of dry kibble, and as meal to be added to wet food. When using commercial food, there are a few rules to observe:

• If you use canned food, add some dry kibble (⅔ wet food to ⅓ meal) to prevent tartar buildup on teeth.
• If the can comes straight from the refrigerator, add a little hot water, otherwise the dog may get diarrhea.
• If you use dry food, make sure the dog has plenty of fresh drinking water available.

Even though commercial dog food offers a well-balanced diet, your dog will enjoy a meal prepared especially for it now and then. Instructions on preparing your own food are on page 15.

Eating Place and Feeding Times

We don't like to be bothered when we eat; neither does your dog. Put its food and water dishes in a spot it can get at any time of day or night and where it can eat without interruptions.

Feed the dog at set times it can get used to. An adult dog should get its main meal around noon and a small snack in the evening. If these times are inconvenient for you, you can give the main meal in the morning or early evening. But whatever time you decide on, make sure that the dog has a short walk 4 to 6 hours after eating to relieve itself.

Drinking Is Important

A dog should always have fresh water available. Dogs should not drink milk on a regular basis because it tends to cause diarrhea if it's undiluted. Old dogs tend not to drink enough. If your dog refuses to drink water but likes milk, offer it a mixture of half skim or buttermilk and half water, but be sure to check for signs of diarrhea.

Bones

Having things to chew on is important for keeping a dog's teeth healthy. Especially if its diet consists primarily of soft, commercial food, the dog should be given rawhide bones, milk bones, or meat bones.

Don't give your dog meat bones more often than twice a week. The best kind are the ball part of ball-and-socket joints from veal or beef. Poultry

bones, pork bones, and hollow leg bones can splinter easily and can cause serious injuries in the digestive tract, such as intestinal puncture or blockage of the intestine (see page 46). Any bone you give your dog should be carefully examined and discarded if it begins to splinter or spoil. Meat bones spoil easily in warm weather.

The Diet of a Puppy

Puppies need a diet that is richer in proteins and minerals than that for full-grown dogs. That is why manufacturers sell special dog food for puppies. If you are getting a puppy, ask the previous owner to give you some of the food the puppy has been getting. This will be helpful while the puppy adjusts to its new home. Consult with your veterinarian regarding the suitability of any diet for your breed of dog.

A puppy should be fed according to the following schedule:
• 3 meals a day until age 3 months;
• 2 meals a day until age 6 months;
• 1 full meal a day thereafter.

The Diet of an Old Dog

Since the liver, kidneys, and intestines don't function as efficiently in old age as they did earlier, an old dog needs food that is high in carbohydrates, which are more easily digested.

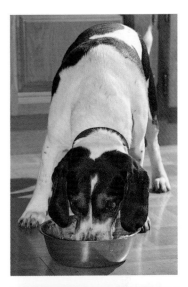

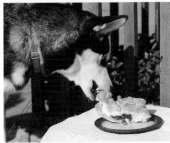

A dog needs to be alone while it is eating. Don't leave a dog unsupervised, however, when there are desserts on the table. Even a well-trained dog can find such a temptation irresistible. This is not only unacceptable behavior but it's also bad for the dog's teeth and general health.

What this means for the menu is less meat and more kibble formulated for older dogs, rice, or vegetables. For certain health conditions, an old dog should get special diet food (see pages 24 and 25). For more information on old dogs, turn to pages 110 to 113.

Improper Diet Gives Rise to Disease

Dogs, like people, have weight problems. In our industrial countries dogs rarely suffer from malnutrition and the deficiency symptoms it causes. Instead, our dogs develop health problems that stem from an overabundance of good food.

Overfeeding often starts when the puppy is still young. Some breeders who want to produce especially strong, large dogs recommend feeding the growing puppy a diet overly high in protein and giving it vitamins and mineral supplements. This can result in abnormal bone growth and joint problems (see pages 88 to 94).

You can check whether your dog is too fat (see drawing) this way: Feel for its ribs behind the shoulder about halfway up the rib cage. The ribs should have only a thin layer of fat over them and should be easy to feel. If you can't feel them, your dog is too fat.

Female dogs are, as a rule, more gluttonous than males, though dogs of both sexes may tend to overeat after they have been neutered. In old dogs that no longer move around a lot weight is often a problem, too. Older dogs especially should be kept in trim shape because excess weight tends to cause joint problems and herniated discs and is also a strain on the heart, lungs, and liver.

Your dog should be put on a diet if it is overweight. Helping it lose weight is a greater proof of love than all the special treats you may be tempted to give it. On page 25 there is a diet designed to help dogs lose weight. If you use commercial dog food you should be aware that the manufacturers tend to err on the generous side in their feeding recommendations. Put less in the dish than the instructions suggest.

Cooking for Your Dog

Dogs like home-made meals cooked especially for them. However, to prevent deficiencies you have to make sure that all the necessary nutritional elements are present in adequate amounts in the food.

Protein is found primarily in meat, fish, and milk products like cottage cheese, though it is also contained in some vegetables, such as soy beans. Essential amino acids are found primarily in proteins of animal origin. The body cannot manufacture them and they therefore have to be provided in the food.

Raw meat is relatively difficult to digest, and consequently should always be cooked first. Pork must never be fed to a dog raw or undercooked because of the danger of toxoplasmosis (see page 101) and of Aujeszky's disease (see Glossary, page 114). Raw poultry meat carries the danger of salmonellosis (see page 100).

Carbohydrates are contained primarily in cereals, kibble, rice, potatoes, and corn. Flour products like pasta, bread, and other baked goods also contain carbohydrates. They are easily digested and, especially if they are made of whole grains, also supply the body with important minerals and vitamins.

Obesity is bad for a dog's health.

Fats are found in meat, especially in pork, and in vegetable oils, and some vegetables, such as corn. Fats are the most abundant source of energy since they contain twice as many calories as carbohydrates and protein. Whether from animal or plant sources, fats and oils contain the so-called fatty acids, some of which the body can't manufacture itself and therefore have to be supplied in the food.

Minerals, trace elements, and vitamins: These are very important, especially for young dogs, but also for old and sick animals. They form part of all the important bodily substances and are contained in the blood, the bones, the muscles, and in other tissues. They are essential for metabolism and for normal and easy movement. If your dog gets dog food enriched with vitamins there is no need to give extra vitamins. Vitamin

and mineral supplements are available from pet stores or from your veterinarian.

The amount of food a dog should get depends on its weight and its individual needs. Other factors to take into account are how much exercise the dog gets and how efficiently its system absorbs the nutrients. The amounts given in the table below are thus meant merely as a guideline.

Home-made Dog Food

Daily need	60% protein	30% carbohydrates	5–10% fats	Vitamins, minerals, trace elements
Small dog, up to 20 lb (10 kg)	5–7 oz (150–200 g)	2½–3½ oz (75–100 g)	1 tsp oil	¼ tsp
Medium dog, about 40 lb (20 kg)	10–12 oz (300–350 g)	5–7 oz (150–200 g)	2 tsp oil	1 tsp
Large dog, 60 lb (30 kg) or more	17–24 oz (500–700 g)	9–12 oz (250–350 g)	1 tbsp oil	2 tsp

Advice for Dog Owners

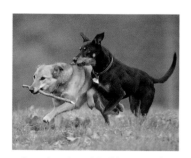

*M*axi and Poldi are eight years old. When their owners picked them up at the breeder's they had no idea of how much they would have to learn in order to take proper care of their pets. But by now they have mastered everything, and the dogs are in perfect shape. You can't find a single lump of matted hair in the dogs' coats, their ears are clean, and their paws are groomed. They look handsome even from behind for their masters don't neglect to clean the area under the tail. If one of the dogs is sick, its owner take its temperature, and knows how to get it to swallow bitter medicine, even if it doesn't want to at all.

Taking the Temperature

A hot, dry nose doesn't mean that a dog has a fever. You can tell a raised temperature only by checking the lower abdomen or the inside of the thighs. If these areas feel unusually warm even when the dog hasn't been exercising you should take the dog's temperature. Use a thin, unbreakable thermometer. The digital kind with a signal tone is best because it reacts more quickly than regular ones. Lubricate the tip with Vaseline. Then hold the standing dog steady (it helps to have two people), lift up its tail, and insert the thermometer, at a slight upward angle, a little over 1 inch (3 cm) into the rectum (see drawing, page 20). The regular old-fashioned thermometers have to be kept in place for 2 to 3 minutes. A digital thermometer can be removed after one minute (after the sound of the signal). If the temperature is above 102.2°F (39°C) in a small dog or above 101.3°F (38.5°C) in a big dog, this has to be considered a fever. A temperature that is below normal (below 100.4°F or 38°C) can also be a sign of illness.

Taking the Pulse

If you suspect that your dog may be sick, you should also check its pulse. The best place to feel the pulse is in the middle of the thigh on the inside. If you use the tips of your fingers and press lightly, you can feel the pulsing artery in the upper thigh. Depending on the size of the dog, the normal pulse rate is between 70 and 100 beats per minute. Count the number of pulse beats for 15 seconds and multiply by 4. The pulse rate is higher in small dogs than in large ones.

Giving Medicine

Liquid medicines are best given with a plastic syringe without the needle (available from your veterinarian). Insert the syringe into the mouth from the side between the teeth (see drawing, page 30). Tilt the dog's head up slightly, and push the medicine onto the tongue in small amounts, in such a way that the dog has to swallow it.

Pills can be given hidden in a treat, such as a piece of liverwurst or cheese. Watch to make sure the dog doesn't spit the pill out. If this method doesn't work, open the dog's mouth, place the pill far back on the tongue, then hold the mouth shut. Now the dog has no choice but to swallow the "bitter pill." You can insert a little water into the mouth with a syringe to help the pill go down easier.

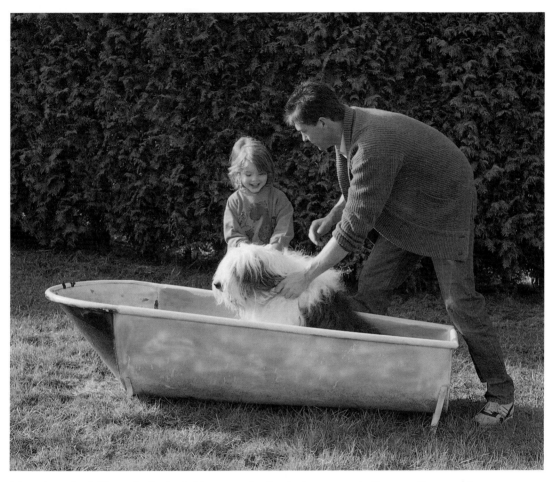

Most dogs don't like to be bathed. However, for hygienic reasons baths sometimes can't be avoided, especially if a dog has gotten extremely dirty or if it has fleas or other parasites.

Putting on a Muzzle

If a dog is in great pain or in shock, it may bite wildly. To be able to help in such a case, you will have to tie the animal's muzzle shut. Take a strong bandage about 3 feet (1 m) long, form a loop with it, and pull the loop over the dog's muzzle. Tighten the loop but not too much, making sure the dog can still breathe through the nose. Then cross the ends of the bandage below the chin and tie them in a bow behind the ears.

HOW-TO: Preventive Care

Grooming for looks is only part of the job. A fashionable clip and a bow on top of the head may be pretty, but regular checking and care of the ears, eyes, teeth, paws, and anus are much more important for the animal's health.

The Coat

If you go about it with a little sensitivity, your dog will interpret grooming as a form of affection.

Brush a short-haired dog once a week, preferably with a brush of natural bristles. Long-haired dogs are first combed with a metal comb with large teeth. Then follow up with a wire brush. Depending on the fineness of the hair, a dog should be combed every day or every other day.

A bath should be given only once a month. Use a non-irritant shampoo (available at pet stores) and be sure to protect the dog's eyes with your hand when you rinse off the shampoo. Or, if you like, you can omit the shampoo and hose the dog down gently every day. Rub the fur well afterwards, use a hair dryer, or let the dog dry in a warm room to keep it from catching cold.

Important: When you brush the coat, check for parasites and for changes in the skin, such as scabby, purulent or red places (see pages 80–84). Pet stores and veterinarians sell flea combs that are fine enough to remove fleas and flea dirt from the coat.

Badly matted fur can give rise to eczema, involving the underlying skin. That is why you should try to gently disentangle the matted hair with your fingers. If the knots don't yield to your fingers, you have to cut them out with scissors, but do it very carefully. In order not to injure the skin, push the blade with the blunt tip into the matted hair first, and don't lift up the skin when you cut. Also make sure there is only hair and no skin between the tips of the scissors.

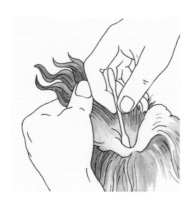

1. Introduce the Q-tip vertically into the ear.

Ear Care

After the bath or at least once a month you should examine your dog's ears. Look for dirt and redness, or any unusual smell (see page 77). If there is excess ear wax, remove it with a soft tissue moistened with baby oil. If there is a lot of hair inside the ears, you should very carefully pluck the hairs with your fingers (don't use scissors because of the danger of injury). If there is too much hair inside the ears, the ear wax gets stuck in it, predisposing the ear to infection.

You had best have the veterinarian show you how to clean the inside of your dog's ears. A Q-tip has to be inserted into the funnel-shaped ear cavity at a vertical angle (see drawing 1). If you push it in horizontally you may injure the tympanic membrane (eardrum).

Eye Care

Check if any secretion has accumulated in the corners of the eyes and pull the lower eyelid down gently to see if the conjunctiva are red and inflamed (see page 74).

Secretion can be removed with a soft tissue. If it has hardened, first dampen the tissue with lukewarm camomile tea and then carefully soften the dried secretion.

Care of the Teeth

Once every three months you should examine your dog's teeth (see drawing 2). Watch out especially for tartar (see page 40), which shows up as a brownish deposit at the base of the teeth. The gums should not be sore or inflamed. If you find loose or broken teeth or if a foul odor comes from the dog's mouth, you should make an appointment with the veterinarian.

If your dog has periodontal problems, you can brush its teeth regularly. Special toothpaste for dogs is sold by veterinarians and at pet stores.

Care of Paws

If your dog has thickly furred paws, you should cut out the hair between the pads and toes carefully. Otherwise, small

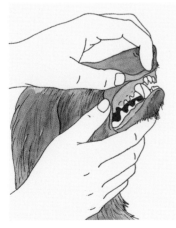

2. Check regularly to see if tartar has formed on the teeth.

stones and things like chewing gum will get stuck in the hair. In the winter, when the dog comes in contact with road salt, it is a good idea to take preventive measures so that the paws don't become inflamed. Rub some Vaseline into the pads and between the toes before you take the dog out, and wash the paws and rubs them dry when you get home again.

Important: If you discover bleeding cracks or cuts in the pads, take the dog to the veterinarian because wounds on the pads often don't heal if left untreated.

Nail Care

A dog that runs enough usually wears its nails down sufficiently. But special "podiatric care" is necessary for older dogs since they are less active and nails grow faster in old age. Small dogs may also need it because less weight means less wear of the nails. Hold up the dog's paw to check the nails' length. If the tip of the nail extends beyond the pad, the nail has to be trimmed (see drawing 3).

It is best to let the veterinarian do the trimming. Part of the nail contains blood vessels and nerves, and it's hard for the untrained to see how far back one can cut safely, especially if the nails are dark.

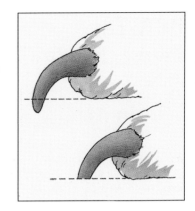

3. Mentally picturing a horizontal line extending from the bottom of the pads helps judge whether the nails are too long.

Care of the Anus and Genital Region

If the area around the dog's anus is sticky and dirty, it is best to hose it down gently or to clean it with a damp cloth. In long-haired dogs the hair around the anus should be cut because secretion from the anal glands and bits of feces often become embedded in it. Dogs try to relieve the itch of a sticky anus by dragging their behinds along the floor or over rugs. This is called "scooting." In young males the hairy tip of the prepuce (foreskin) often gets sticky with pus. In that case the dog has to be taken to the veterinarian who will treat the inflammation with disinfecting and antibiotic solutions.

HOW-TO: Getting Ready To See the Veterinarian

The veterinarian should see your dog not only in situations of acute illness but also for routine preventive care. One regular occasion for a visit to the veterinarian is the annual immunization. At these times the veterinarian should also check the animal's overall state of health. Old dogs should be examined professionally at least twice a year.

Things to Get Ready Before the Visit

In preparation for the trip you should get out the dog's vaccination record and, if you have any, records of previous dewormings. Also take along the medications the dog is receiving, except for those prescribed by the veterinarian. Note down your observations of the dog so you can describe symptoms the dog may have (see pages 4–7). Take a sample of vomit or stool if you have noticed anything unusual in them (blood, worms, foreign bodies). If you have health insurance for your dog (see Glossary, page 116), don't forget to take along the insurance card or other documentation.

The Trip

Most veterinarians make house calls only in exceptional cases. To diagnose illness, technical equipment and trained personnel are generally needed, both of which are available at the office or animal clinic. Since most dogs are used to riding in cars, the trip to the doctor's office is usually unproblematic. In many big cities there are special animal taxis that can be hired to take pets to the veterinarian. Ask at your local animal shelter if such a service is available in your area. If a dog is unable to walk, you will have to carry it in its basket.

Important: A dog that has been in an accident has to be transported with special care. You never know if there are internal injuries or broken bones, and it is therefore important to transport the dog in an immobile position. The best way is to lay the animal on a flat, hard surface such as a board. If nothing like this is available, you can use a blanket on which the dog is carried carefully by two persons (see page 28). In case of an accident, an emergency veterinary service, if available, is helpful.

The Vaccination Schedule

It is extremely important that dogs get vaccinated regularly. A dog without immunization protection is vulnerable to infectious diseases that may be fatal; some of them can be transmitted to humans. Dogs are vaccinated against rabies, distemper, hepatitis, parvovirus, leptospirosis, and sometimes against kennel cough and Lyme disease. Since there is no lifelong immunity to these diseases, the vaccinations have to be repeated annually, for as long as the animal lives.

Puppies are especially vulnerable to disease because their immune system is not yet fully developed. But old dogs are vulnerable, too, and it would be foolish to stop giving a dog its vaccinations from a certain age on.

Keep the vaccination record the veterinarian gives you, and use the most recent date to

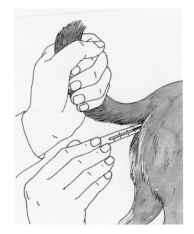

To take the dog's temperature, hold up its tail with one hand and gently introduce the thermometer into the anus.

figure when the next vaccinations are due. Many veterinarians will mail reminder cards a week or two before booster injections are due, so remember to keep your veterinarian updated if you change your address.

Puppies are vaccinated at
• 8 to 9 weeks against distemper, hepatitis, parainfleunza, leptospirosis, and parvovirus (if the kennel had problems with parvovirus, a preliminary vaccination should be given at 5 to 7 weeks);
• 12 to 14 weeks against distemper, hepatitis, leptospirosis, parainfluenza, parvovirus, and rabies. Kennel cough (*Bordetella*) and coronavirus may also be included.

Adult dogs are generally vaccinated annually against: distemper, hepatitis, leptospirosis, parainfluenza, parvovirus, *Bordetella,* and coronavirus; the frequency at which the rabies vaccine is administered (annually or biannually) varies, depending on the recommendation of your veterinarian.

Deworming
Regular fecal examination for parasites and deworming is important for two reasons. First, an animal weakened by worms is more susceptible to infections, and, second, worms can be transmitted to humans. Children, especially, risk getting worms from dogs (see Parasites, page 101).

Dogs should be dewormed at
• 6 weeks;
• 8 weeks (preceding the first vaccination);
• 12 weeks (preceding the second vaccination);
• 6 months;
• 9 months.

Adult dogs should be dewormed twice a year. If your dog has fleas or digs often after mice, it should be dewormed more often. The most common tapeworm in dogs is transmitted by fleas. Since there are different kinds of worms (see pages 101, 102), a worm medicine effective against a broad spectrum of worms should be used. Ask your veterinarian for advice.

Important: Dewormings should always be performed before immunization so that the dog is in full health when it is vaccinated.

What the Veterinarian Needs to Know
For the veterinarian to be able to diagnose and treat a sick dog he or she must have as much and as detailed information from you as possible. Jot down what you have observed, including how long the dog has shown symptoms, how they manifest themselves (for example body posture when in pain, kind of cough), and the situations in which they occur. The following check list shows you some basic questions.

Check List
Make note of the following:
• When and what did the dog last eat and drink?
• When did it last pass urine and stools? Did it have difficulty doing so?
• What was the consistency of the stools? (Take along a sample.) Was there blood in the urine?
• Did the dog vomit? How often and what? How long after last feeding? (Take along a sample.)
• Is there bloating or are there rumbling noises from the intestines? Is gas being passed from the anus?
• Has the dog been sneezing, coughing, drooling, or choking?
• Does it have a fever? (see page 16) How high is the temperature?
• Is the dog limping or lame? When did it start? In what situation?
• Does the dog stand with arched back, or does it walk stiffly?
• Does it have difficulty getting up?
• Does it stop in front of stairs or refuse to jump into the car?
• Does it lick, scratch, or bite itself in some parts of the body?
• Does it drag its rear end along the ground and try to lick its tail?
• Does it often shake its head and scratch its ears?
• Does touching certain parts of its body cause it pain?

HOW-TO: Taking Care of a Sick Dog

The veterinarian has made a diagnosis and decided on a course of treatment. Perhaps surgery is necessary, and perhaps you will have to care for your pet at home over a prolonged period. In order to regain its health or to live comfortably in spite of a chronic condition your pet will need your help.

Getting Ready for Anesthesia
Anesthesia is required not only for surgery. A sedation or light anesthesia is also often administered for things like cleaning tartar off the teeth, irrigating the ears, keeping the animal from feeling pain, or simply to keep it from moving.

You have to prepare your dog for anesthesia: It should not get anything to eat during the preceding 12 hours, though it is allowed to drink water for up to 6 hours before anesthesia.

Important: For major surgery (neutering, removal of a tumor, or operating on bones), the dog should be bathed beforehand to minimize the danger of infection.

Postoperative Care
Usually an animal that has undergone surgery is not allowed to return home until all risk is past and it is conscious again, though still tired and groggy. Old and obese animals remain unconscious longer. You should observe the following rules if you take your dog home before it has regained consciousness:

• To make sure that the dog doesn't get cold, cover it with a blanket both during the trip and when you get home. Or shine an infrared heat lamp on it; to prevent thermal burns in your pet, never use a heating pad.
• Open the mouth and pull the tongue out so that the dog can't choke on it.
• Check the breathing. The dog should take a breath every 5 to 8 seconds.
• Check the pulse (see page 16).
Important: A dog should not eat anything for 12 hours after

Dogs that pull on a bandage have to wear an Elizabethan collar.

an operation, but you can let it drink after 6 hours.

Care of Incision
Veterinarians generally don't bandage minor incisions in order for the air to get at them and speed up healing. The incision does have to be bandaged if there is reason to think that the dog will lick it. An incision that is not bandaged should be dabbed dry 2 or 3 times a day with a tissue or some cotton. If a drain (see Glossary, page 116) was installed, dabbing will be necessary more frequently. After dabbing the incision, apply a healing spray or powder only if prescribed by the veterinarian.

Important: Don't use any ointments. They may soften the scab that is trying to form.

Changing a Bandage
Depending on how much the wound oozes, a change of bandage may be necessary anywhere from twice a day to every other day. For changing the bandage you need a compress—drug stores sell sterile gauze packs—and a fresh bandage. Place the sterile gauze on the incision after dabbing it clean (see above) and then wrap the bandage not too tightly around the affected part of the body.

A body bandage: If a dog has to have its body bandaged, you can buy a tubular bandage (available at drugstores) or fashion one yourself out of an old T-shirt or pantyhose (see photo, page 80). Before applying a body bandage, consult your veterinarian.

Important: Don't use band-aids on wounds. The skin under the adhesive part will get sore, and when you pull the bandaid off, the hairs and sometimes some skin are torn off.

An Elizabethan Collar

If your dog rips off all bandages, you may have to put an Elizabethan collar on it at night or when you can't watch it. Your veterinarian can supply you with one of these funnel-shaped devices (see drawing, page 22).

Insulin Injections

If your dog has diabetes you will have to give it insulin shots once or twice a day to lower the blood sugar. (The veterinarian will give you syringes with needles.) Find a place where the skin is loose (the neck, back, or the side of the body), pull it up with three fingers into a kind of tent shape, and then stick the needle into the empty space below the tent top. Let go of the skin, make sure the tip of the needle is below the skin but hasn't penetrated anywhere else. Now push down the plunger of the syringe with the hand that held up the skin fold.

Important: Pick a new place for each injection.

Inhalation

If the veterinarian has prescribed inhalation therapy for your dog, heat some camomile extract (available at health food stores); Vick's Vaporub or Mentholatum or prescribed drug, and water in a saucepan and drape a cover over it tent-fashion. Now try to get the dog to hold its head under the cover so that it will inhale the vapors. Not many dogs put up with this.

You will have better luck using an inhalator that works by means of ultrasound. These inhalators can be obtained from drug stores or companies specializing in medical equipment. The dog inhales the vapors and medications through a kind of funnel (see drawing, page 55).

Medicated Baths

Be very sparing in your use of medicinal shampoos (obtained from the veterinarian or bought at pet stores). Don't forget that shampoos effective against fleas and other parasites contain insecticides, that is, potentially toxic substances if used in excess.
• Protect the dog's eyes by putting ointment on them and placing some cotton moistened with oil in the ears before you shampoo the dog.
• Let the lathered shampoo work for 5 to 10 minutes before rinsing it off well with clear water. Then rub the dog dry.

Important: Make sure the dog doesn't lap up any of the bath water. And wash your hands thoroughly once you have finished. If you have sensitive skin or tend to develop allergic reactions you should wear disposable rubber gloves (see Important Notes, page 127).

Rubbing Medication into the Skin

If a dog suffers from skin problems, such as ringworm or mange (see pages 81, 82), it is often necessary to shave the dog and treat the entire body. There are several proprietary and prescription parasiticidal medications available that can be safely applied to the entire body of the dog. Consult your veterinarian.

Important: Wash your hands well after applying the ointment (see above).

Eye Drops and Ointments

Applying eye drops: Pull the lower eyelid slightly away from the eye, and place 2 to 3 drops inside the lid.

Applying eye ointment: Lift the upper eyelid a little and squeeze a strip of ointment ¼ to ½ inch (5–10 mm) long under the lid.

HOW-TO: Diets for Sick Dogs

In addition to medication, a special diet is often required as well. In some cases, as with chronic kidney, liver, and pancreas conditions (see pages 66, 50, 51), diabetes (see page 87), and food allergies, a dog may have to stay on a special diet for the rest of its life. Information on the various nutritional elements is given on pages 14 and 15. Your dog's veterinarian can advise you on specific diets, and usually has commercially prepared products you can buy.

Diet for Gastrointestinal Disorders

Gastrointestinal disorders are generally accompanied by vomiting and diarrhea. That is why a dog should fast for one day before starting on the diet and on this day be given or made to swallow small amounts of sweetened black tea instead of water.

The diet has to be
• high in carbohydrates (about 70%)
• low in protein (about 30%); and
• very low in fat.
  The ideal recipe:
• 70% cooked oatmeal or rice

made appetizing by the addition of meat stock;
• 30% chopped chicken;
• 1 teaspoon vegetable oil per 20 pounds (10 kg) body weight;
• ½ teaspoon vitamin and mineral supplement per 20 pounds (10 kg) body weight if the diet has to be continued over a long period.
  Important: Divide the food into 3 to 4 small portions and

Food Amounts in Special Diets
The amount of food depends on the individual needs of the dog and varies depending on age, amount of exercise, and, above all, how well the animal absorbs the nutrients. The following is only a rough guideline.
• Total daily amount: 9 ounces (250 g) of food per 20 pounds (10 kg) body weight.

give them in the course of the day. The dog can be given sweetened black tea to drink.
  Commercial diet dog food for gastrointestinal disorders is sold by veterinarians.

Kidney Diet
The kidneys filter nitrogenous wastes out of the blood, substances that become toxic if they stay in the body. A protein-rich diet made up mostly of meat puts a special strain on the kidneys.
  Make the diet
• low in protein (10 to 20%);

• high in carbohydrates (70 to 80%); and
• low in fat (up to 10%).
  The ideal recipe:
• 20% poached or sauteed fish;
• 80% cooked rice or mashed potatoes;
• 1 teaspoon vegetable oil;
• 2 to 3 grams table salt per 20 lb (10 kg) body weight.
  Salt is necessary for the functioning of the kidneys and always has to be present in the food. Dogs with kidney problems may have an increased need for salt.
  Important: If a dog is also suffering from heart disease, salt intake must be reduced.
  Commercial diet dog food for kidney problems is sold by veterinarians.

Liver Diet
Especially in the case of chronic liver disease (see page 50), an easily digestible diet is important. The diet should not impose unnecessary effort on the liver, assist in its regeneration, and reduce the fat in the liver tissue.
  The diet should be
• high in carbohydrates (75%);
• low in protein (25%); and
• almost completely fat-free.
  The ideal recipe:
• 25% low-fat or fat-free cottage cheese;
• 75% cooked rice, cream of wheat, or oatmeal;
• glucose sugar, honey, or jam as sweetener;
• 1 teaspoon vegetable oil per 20 pounds (10 kg) body weight;

- ½ teaspoon vitamin and mineral supplement per 20 pounds (10 kg) body weight.

Important: Sweet things don't harm a dog's teeth as long as the dog gets plenty of opportunity to chew. Supply stale bread, rawhide bones, and meat bones, especially ball joints.

As a ready-made diet food you can use the special diet dog food for gastrointestinal problems sold by veterinarians and add 10% food meal. Check with your veterinarian before modifying any prescription diet.

Pancreas Diet

The ingredients of a diet for a malfunctioning pancreas have to be
- rich in easily digestible proteins (60%);
- fairly low in carbohydrates (30%); and
- low in fat.

The ideal recipe:
- 60% lean beef or pork (never feed the meat raw), which will include the required fat;
- 30% mashed potatoes, cooked rice, or noodles;
- beef pancreas (available from the butcher or from slaughter houses) or pancreas powder (available from the veterinarian); the amount depends on the seriousness of the condition.

Important: For the food to be better digested, mix it with the chopped pancreas tissue or the powder and keep it in the refrigerator for one day or let it stand at room temperature for 4 hours.

Weight Loss Diet

Dogs that have been neutered or that suffer from hormonal imbalances are often compulsive eaters and wolf down anything they find. To help them feel less hungry you should give them food that is high in fiber and roughage.

The ideal recipe:
- 50% cooked vegetables of all kinds (except potatoes) as a substitute for carbohydrates;
- 25% bran, alfalfa hay meal, or dried beet chips (available at health food stores);
- 25% tripe, or lung in place of regular meat;
- 1 teaspoon vegetable oil per 20 pounds (10 kg) body weight;
- ½ teaspoon vitamin and mineral supplement per 20 pounds (10 kg) body weight.

Important: Use lean meat and fat-free milk products.

Commercial weight loss diet food for dogs (both dry and canned) is available from your veterinarian or at pet stores.

The fermenting agents in the pancreas tissue start breaking down the food before it is eaten. Divide the daily amount into 3 or 4 portions and feed them over the course of the day.

As a ready-made diet you can use the commercial diet dog food for gastrointestinal problems (available from the veterinarian) and add 20% lean meat.

Diet for Diabetes

Diabetic dogs nevertheless need sugar (carbohydrates) in their food. A diet based entirely on meat (protein) causes kidney problems and vitamin and mineral deficiency symptoms.

The diet should have
- 60 or 70% protein;
- 20 or 30% carbohydrates;
- 5 or 10% fat (diabetics also can't metabolize fats normally).

The ideal recipe:
See Pancreas Diet.

Important: The following feeding schedule seems to work well: 3 feedings given 4 to 6 hours apart with the amount being decreased by about half each time.

As a ready-made diet you can use the special diet for gastrointestinal problems (available from the veterinarian) and add 20% meat.

Diet for Allergies

To find out what the dog is allergic to, feed it as neutral a diet and as unlikely a one to cause allergies as possible.

The ideal recipe:
- 50% lamb, poultry, or cottage cheese;
- 50% cooked rice.

Important: Continue with the diet for one week, until the symptoms disappear. Then reintroduce the elements of the original diet one by one to find out which has caused the allergy.

Commercial diets for allergic dogs are available from the vet.

HOW-TO: What to Do in Case of Accidents

It can happen if you fail to watch for even one moment: Your dog runs across the street and is hit by a car even though the driver slammed on the brakes. What kind of injuries the dog sustains depends on what part of the dog's body is hit and also on what part of the car it collides with.

Injuries result not only from car accidents but often from dog fights as well. Dogs can inflict serious bite wounds on each other.

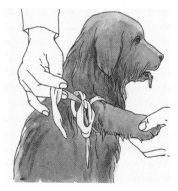

1. Put a tourniquet on the leg above the elbow or the heel.

Emergency Measures after an Accident

First try to calm your dog by talking to it gently. Then try to get a sense of how seriously it got hurt by examining it very carefully.

• Stopping the Bleeding
Especially if the blood spurts out with every beat of the pulse you'll have to stop the bleeding quickly with a tourniquet. Tie the tourniquet on the leg above the heel or the elbow (see drawing 1). If you don't have a regular tourniquet, you can use a stocking or sock. It is important for the material to be elastic. The tourniquet has to be loosened for 30–60 seconds every 20–30 minutes to let blood flow into the limb; otherwise the limb might necrose. If the bleeding involves a bigger area, a pressure dressing has to be applied (see drawing, page 27).

• Keeping the Airways Open
If a dog loses consciousness you have to make sure it can still breathe freely. Open the muzzle and make sure the airway is not obstructed. Any vomit that may be there has to be removed. Then pull the tongue out somewhat and lay it between the side teeth.

• Protect Yourself Against Injury
Don't reach for the dog spontaneously after an accident. Dogs may bite—even their owners—if they are in pain or in shock after an accident. If, for example, you have to put on a temporary bandage (see First Aid, page 128), you'll want first to tie the dog's muzzle shut (see page17). But make sure the nose is left uncovered.

• Taking the Dog to the Vet
After these emergency measures are taken, you'll need to take the dog to the veterinarian as quickly as possible. You can use a blanket as a kind of stretcher (see drawing, page 28). If you suspect injury to the spine, a board or some other flat and rigid object should be placed under the blanket for support (see also page 128).

Traumatic Shock

Dogs are usually in a state of shock after being in an accident. In this state the vital organs receive insufficient blood and oxygen.

Symptoms: Pale mucous membranes, racing pulse, fast breathing, below-normal temperature, listlessness, loss of consciousness.

First aid: First make sure the dog is resting comfortably on its side, covered with a blanket, breathing freely, and getting enough fresh air. Then rush it to the veterinarian. When given plenty of oxygen, drugs to stimulate the circulation, and intravenous fluids, a dog usually recovers from traumatic shock within an hour.

Air in the Pleural Cavity

If something hits the dog in the area of the rib cage, small tears in the lungs may result. Air is pressed out through these tears into the pleural cavity and keeps the lungs from expanding fully (pneumothorax).

A blow to the abdominal area can lead to a torn diaphragm (see page 58).

Symptoms: Pumping breathing, pale blue mucous membranes.

First aid: Make sure the dog can breathe freely (see page 26). Place it sitting up (perhaps supported by a pillow or rolled up blankets). Then take it to the veterinarian.

Injuries to the Chest Wall

The chest wall can be punctured by sharp objects or by broken ribs.

Symptoms: With each breath air "hisses" out of the wound.

First aid: Cover wound immediately with a clean cloth or a compress, put on a pressure bandage, and bandage the entire rib cage (see drawing 2) to close the wound as tightly as possible. Otherwise the condition may develop into pneumothorax or pleurisy (see page 57). Take the animal to the veterinarian.

Internal Abdominal Injuries

The impact of blunt objects on the abdominal area can result in contusions severe enough to cause tearing of the tissue of internal organs, such as the spleen, liver, intestines, bladder, and kidneys.

• If the spleen, liver, or kidneys are injured there is usually heavy bleeding into the abdominal cavity.

Symptoms: Pale mucous membranes, rapid pulse, pain in the belly, general drastic decline within minutes or hours.

Important: If you notice the mucous membranes of your dog turning pale—even if there is no external sign of injury—take the animal to the veterinarian immediately.

• If there are tears in the intestines or the bladder without

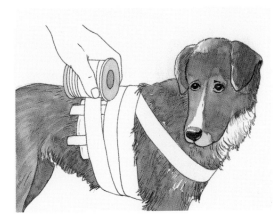

2. Hold a chest bandage in place by wrapping an elastic ace bandage around the body and across the shoulders. Attach the bandage securely with adhesive tape.

major bleeding, there is some initial pain in the belly area, but no clear symptoms appear until 1 to 3 days after the accident. These symptoms are caused by advancing peritonitis (see page 51) and toxemia.

Symptoms: High fever, apathy, very painful belly, vomiting.

Important: Take the animal to the veterinarian as quickly as you can. With the aid of X-rays

27

and contrast media that show up the intestines and bladder, the veterinarian can arrive at a precise diagnosis and, if surgery can be initiated in time, save your dog.

Concussion

In severe head trauma a concussion may be associated with swelling of the brain, called cerebral edema, which results in malfunctionings of the central nervous system.

Symptoms: Dazed state, wobbliness, shaking the head, trembling of the eyes, uneven dilation of the pupils, excessive salivating, vomiting, epileptic seizures (fits).

First aid: Make sure the dog is resting comfortably in an absolutely quiet place. Calm the animal if necessary, and keep its airways clear (see page 26). Be careful to avoid being bitten. Put a blanket over the dog to keep it from getting cold. See the veterinarian as soon as possible.

Spinal Injuries

The vertebral column protects the spinal cord within the spinal canal. Vertebrae fractured in an accident or a fall can lead to contusion or severing of the spinal cord.

Symptoms: Pain and cramping in the back, paralysis, loss of sensation in the legs.

Important: If you suspect spinal injuries, rush the dog to the veterinarian instantly. Be especially careful in transporting the animal (see pages 26 and 128).

Fractures, Dislocations, and Ligament Injuries

Accidents and falls often cause fractures. If the skin over the broken bone remains intact, we speak of a closed fracture. If the bone protrudes through the skin, this is a "compound" fracture, which can easily become infected.

When a bone is pushed out of its joint, we speak of a dislocated joint. In ligament injuries, the ligaments and muscles have been stretched and partially or completely torn. These conditions are hard to tell apart from simple fractures.

Symptoms: A cracking noise on movement of the injured limb, painful limping even if no weight is put on the limb, swelling, change of shape, buckling near the injury; the broken bone may be exposed.

First aid: Put a muzzle restraint on the dog if necessary (see page 17) so that you won't be bitten. Move the affected leg as little as possible. You may want to stabilize it with a temporary splint (page 129). Lay the dog down as gently and comfortably as possible, supporting it with a rolled up blanket, and spread another blanket over it for warmth. If the bone is exposed, cover it with a clean cloth to reduce the danger of infection. Take the dog to the veterinarian immediately.

Healing of bones: Fractures can heal most readily only if the broken parts are joined together again as perfectly as possible and if the affected limb is kept from moving.

• A fracture is immobilized for at least 3 to 6 weeks with the help of bandages and a splint (of aluminum or moldable

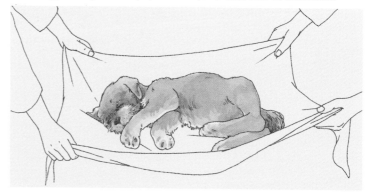

1. If there is no board or other hard, flat surface available, a dog that was injured in a car accident can be carried on a blanket.

plastic). But this works only for broken ribs and certain types of fractures of the bones below the elbow and the knee. The bandage has to be changed and the fracture checked once a week.

• All fractures that are not treated with a splint are repaired surgically. Internal bone fixation, as it is called (see Glossary, page 117), is used especially if a fracture is near a joint or if there are small splinters. To hold the bones in place, wires, hollow nails, screws, or metal plates are used. These implants usually have to be removed after 3 to 6 months.

• Surgery for torn ligaments and dislocated joints: Torn ligaments and damage to the socket, which are unavoidable in dislocated joints, have to be fixed by suturing or, quite often, by replacing a ligament (especially in the knee).

Bite Wounds

Dogs that are excessively aggressive frequently get bitten. You should therefore look your dog over carefully after any dog fight. Otherwise, wounds may remain undetected in a thick coat and may develop abscesses if an opponent's teeth have broken the skin.

First aid: If your dog has sustained a wound that bleeds, the wound should be covered with a clean cloth. If the blood is spurting out, put on a pressure

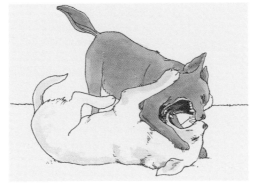

bandage or, in an emergency, exert pressure on the blood vessel with your hand so that the dog will not bleed to death. Then take the animal to the veterinarian immediately.

In order to prevent infections, the veterinarian has to open the wound more to remove hair and dirt that may have been embedded there by the rival's teeth, and a drain has to be installed for the fluid secretions from the wound to flow off.

Important: Sometimes an abscess doesn't form until several days after the fight. Then it causes fever, apathy, loss of appetite, and blood poisoning. Therefore, you should take your dog to the veterinarian if it has any bite wound.

Burns

Burns are most often caused by scalding with hot water or oil or by contact with a hot surface (an oven door or stove burner). If the fur gets wet with some

2. Check your dog all over for bite wounds after every dog fight it gets into. If there are any wounds, have the veterinarian look at them.

caustic substance, burns can also result.

Symptoms: The skin is red and painful when touched, or discolored to a whitish or brown color; the hair in the affected place is singed or missing; blisters form, with the skin underneath red and shriveled.

First aid: Cool the burn wound quickly under cold, running water or place an ice bag on it. The water helps in case of a caustic burn by diluting and rinsing away the irritating substance. If the deeper layers of the skin are affected, cover the wound with a clean cloth or bandage and take the animal to the veterinarian right away.

HOW-TO: First Aid in Cases of Poisoning

Poisons are substances that cause severe, abnormal reactions in the body and may even lead to death. We—and consequently our dogs—encounter poisons in different forms, as in rat poison, medications, insecticides, and disinfectants. Dog owners and, unfortunately, veterinarians as well are too often satisfied to ascribe certain conditions to undefined poisoning. You should assume that you're dealing with a case of poisoning only if there are unmistakable symptoms. Many other disorders can exhibit symptoms that resemble those of poisoning. If, however, you have seen your dog eat or come in contact with something toxic, take it to the veterinarian immediately. Don't wait for the first signs of poisoning. The earlier counter measures are initiated (evacuation and rinsing out the stomach, giving antidotes), the better the chance that the dog can be helped. If you know what poison your pet was exposed to, have the information from the label available for the veterinarian.

Preventive Measures

There are ways to minimize the chance of poisoning.

Watch on walks and make sure your dog doesn't eat anything. Puppies in particular tend to gobble up all kinds of things.

• Keep an eye out in public places for signs that mouse or rat poisons are being used. Don't take your dog walking there or don't let if off the leash.

• Remove all poisonous plants from your home or place them where the dog can't get at them.

• Lock up all chemicals, cleaning agents, insecticides, and medications. Don't forget antifreeze and rat and mouse poisons.

• When giving your dog flea baths and especially when using sprays, make sure the animal doesn't absorb too much of the insecticide (see Glossary, page 117).

Main Symptoms of Poisoning

Excessive salivation; repeated vomiting and sometimes diarrhea; blood in the vomit, stool, or urine; apathy; shortness of breath; pale or bluish mucous membranes; racing pulse; staggering; convulsions; loss of consciousness, change in pupil size.

If the symptoms occur within 1 or 2 hours and in the order in which they are listed above, the dog is most likely suffering from poisoning.

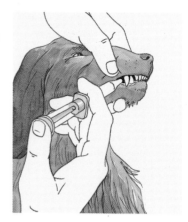

If your dog has ingested poison, introduce a strong salt solution into its mouth with a syringe.

Emergency Measures

Emetics, stomach and intestinal rinses, and laxatives help get poisons out of the system only if they are administered within half an hour to an hour after the poison was ingested.

• Take the dog to the veterinarian immediately.

• If the nearest veterinarian is some distance away, try to induce vomiting—after consulting with the veterinarian by phone—by force feeding (see drawing) the dog a concentrated saline solution (1 tablespoon salt in 3 ounces [100 ml] water) and medication (see page 16). Some areas also have a poison control hotline that you can call for advice. Keep this number with your list of emergency telephone numbers.

Important: Never make the dog drink milk, oil, and

especially not castor oil because in the case of some fat soluble poisons this would aggravate the condition.

• Give the dog tablets of activated charcoal. Charcoal absorbs most poisons and is not harmful to the animal.

• Give the dog plenty to drink. Water has a diluting effect and acts almost like a stomach rinse if the dog vomits after drinking.

The Most Common Causes of Poisoning

In the case of some poisons there are symptoms that will quickly give you a clue as to what caused the poisoning. Then take the dog to the veterinarian immediately.

• **Antifreeze** (ethylene glycol): If your dog licks up sweet tasting antifreeze, it may develop severe kidney damage and—depending on the amount of poison consumed—complete kidney failure. Antifreeze toxicity often results in death, so prevention of exposure to this poison is essential.

Symptoms: Excessive salivation, spontaneous vomiting within minutes after absorbing the antifreeze, diarrhea, listlessness, staggering, convulsions, general weakness.

Treatment: Stomach rinses, infusions to keep the kidneys working; as an antidote ethyl alcohol is used intravenously.

• **Sleeping pills** (barbiturates): If a dog eats sleeping tablets, this will result in a state similar to

Insecticides

(Organophosphates, carbamates, chlorinated hydrocarbons)

If substances intended to combat feas, lice, and ticks (in the form of shampoos, powders, sprays, a flea/tick collar, tablets, or tinctures) are not handled properly, the dog can poison itself if, for instance, it licks its fur after too heavy a powdering or spraying, drinks the bath water (see page 23), chews on the collar, or swallows too many tablets.

Symptoms: Insecticides are nerve toxins and give rise to symptoms similar to those of poisoning with snail bait (see right-hand column).

Treatment: As for poisoning with metaldehyde (see right-hand column).

Important: After powdering the dog, wipe the coat with a damp bath towel; after shampooing, rinse well; and be sure not to leave flea collars lying around.

anesthesia or possibly death will result.

Symptoms: No vomiting or diarrhea; deep sleep; loss of consciousness; shallow breathing; bluish mucous membranes; fast, weak pulse.

Treatment: Administer emetics and stomach rinses; artificial respiration with oxygen, infusions to stimulate the circulatory system so that the kidneys will start eliminating the

poisons. The dog has to be kept warm while it is asleep and should be moved or rotated to a different position every half hour to prevent the blood from stagnating in internal organs, especially the lungs.

• **Rat poison:** Rodenticides containing coumarin or warfarin sodium are poisons that interfere with blood clotting.

Symptoms: At first some minor vomiting that is often overlooked; after 2 to 6 days listlessness caused by internal bleeding; pale mucous membranes; very bloody urine and sometimes bloody diarrhea.

Treatment: Vitamin K1 injections as an antidote and perhaps blood transfusion.

• **Metaldehyde** (used as snail and slug bait and as a smokeless fuel): The dog eats the snail bait in the garden or cubes of the fuel it finds in the house. This nerve poison can, depending on the amount ingested, lead to death within 24 hours.

Symptoms: Excessive salivation after half an hour to an hour, vomiting, diarrhea. After another 1 to 3 hours, incoordination; staggering; nervousness; stiff, straddling legs (even when lying down); cramp attacks with stretched head; high fever (105.8 to 107.6°F [41–42°C]).

Treatment: Emetics, stomach rinses, sedatives and barbiturates that induce a healing sleep for 1 to 2 days. Intravenous fluids to stimulate the kidneys; calcium to alleviate cramps.

HOW-TO: A Small Medical Kit for the Dog

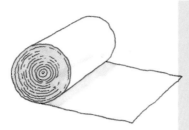

You should always have a small supply of medications, bandaging materials, and a few instruments on hand to take care of cuts, bites, and other minor wounds, as well as for preventive and follow-up care. Whether you also want to prepare a special first aid kit for the dog is up to you.

The following list of things is meant only as a suggestion and makes no claim to completeness. Consult with your veterinarian. He or she will recommend other medications if, for example, you plan to take a major trip with your dog (see also Imported Diseases, pages 102 and 103). It is a good idea to keep emergency numbers, such as the phone numbers of your veterinarian and a poison control center, in this kit for ready access.

Bandaging Materials
• 2 or 3 gauze rolls 1½ or 2½ inches (4 or 6 cm) wide for bandaging paws;
• 2 or 3 gauze rolls 3 to 4 inches (8–10 cm) wide for bandaging head, chest, or abdomen;
• 1 small package gauze pads;
• 1 heavy bandage for tying the muzzle shut and for tying off a bleeding limb;
• 1 roll adhesive tape 2½ inches (6 cm) wide;
• 1 roll adhesive tape 1 inch (2.5 cm) wide;
• 1 package cotton balls or loose cotton;
• 1 box tissues;
• 1 box Q-tips.

Disinfectants
• 1 small bottle (½ ounce or 20 ml) antiseptic tincture (for example, mercurochrome or povidone-iodine solution);
• 1 small bottle (½ ounce or 20 ml) hydrogen peroxide (3%) solution for dabbing on inflamed gums;
• 1 larger bottle (3 ounces or 100 ml) isopropyl alcohol (70%) to rub in as a coolant and for disinfecting instruments.

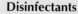
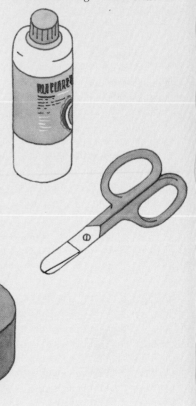

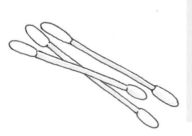

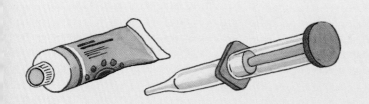

• 1 pair surgical tweezers with rounded points;
• 2 or 3 wooden tongue depressors for applying ointments;
• 1 syringe each of 2 ml, 5 ml, and 10 ml size (without the needles) for giving liquids, food, or medications.

Ointments and Liquids
• 1 jar or tube healing ointment (for example, Betadine, Nolvasan, Desitin)
• 1 small bottle diethyl ether for cleaning up and for removing adhesive tape;
• 1 small bottle eye drops to relieve itching (for example, Visine, Murine, Dacriose Ophthalmic Irrigating Solution);
• 1 bottle baby oil for cleaning the ears;
• 1 jar Vaseline for paw care.

Medications You Should Keep on Hand
• Activated charcoal against diarrhea. Dogs get one tablet twice a day per 20 pounds (10 kg) body weight.
• Vitamin and mineral supplements (in powder or tablet form) to be added to the food especially for puppies and sick dogs. Ask your veterinarian for advice.
Important: Keep track of the expiration date of the medica-

tions. Don't use drugs past the date stamped on them. Return them to the drugstore because they should be disposed of as hazardous waste.

Instruments
• 1 rectal thermometer (either a regular, unbreakable one or a plastic one with digital indicator);
• 1 pair curved scissors with one pointed and one blunt blade;
• 1 pair scissors for cutting bandages;
• 1 pair tweezers for removing ticks;

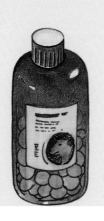

For Special Conditions
• If your dog is diabetic, you have to have insulin and special insulin syringes and needles for the daily injections (keep it in the refrigerator). You should also have a bottle of corn syrup handy in case of hypoglycemic

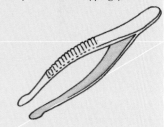

shock. Ask your veterinarian how much to administer.
• There are powders, sprays, and shampoos against fleas, lice, ticks, and other parasites of the skin (see pages 81 and 82). Keep them on hand for when they are needed.
Important: Use all these substances with great caution (see Important Notes, page 127). A useful book for emergency situations is *First Aid for Your Dog* by Frederic Frye, Barron's, 1987.

33

Recognizing and Treating

1. Skull
2. Maxilla
3. Mandible
4. Cervical vertebrae
5. Scapula
6. Shoulder joint
7. Humerus
8. Elbow joint
9. Radius and ulna
10. Metacarpals
11. Carpals
12. Rib cage
13. Stifle (knee) joint
14. Metatarsals
15. Hock joint and heel
16. Tibia and fibula
17. Femur
18. Hip joint
19. Coccygeal vertebrae (tail)
20. Pelvis
21. Thoracic and lumbar vertebrae

Skeleton of a Dog

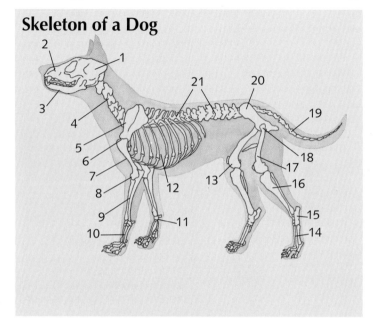

1. Oral cavity
2. Tongue
3. Windpipe or trachea
4. Heart
5. Liver
6. Spleen
7. Small intestine
8. Penis
9. Testicle
10. Spermatic cord
11. Colon
12. Bladder
13. Ureter
14. Kidneys
15. Stomach
16. Lung
17. Esophagus
18. Larynx

Internal Organs of a Dog

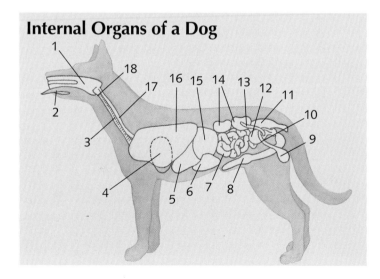

Dog Diseases

The causes of illness are many. Heat, cold, exposure to dampness, pathogens like bacteria, fungi, viruses, and parasites, and environmental factors are all external causes. Diseases can also be inherited, and we speak of psychological illness if, for instance, a dog is depressed when left alone.

The healing process is essentially accomplished by the body itself through its resistance and regenerative powers. Medicine is only the handmaiden of nature and of the body's power to heal itself. This principle lies at the heart of homeopathic medicine.

Depending on the course an illness takes we distinguish between acute diseases (which appear suddenly) and chronic ones (gradual and lingering). The veterinarian examines the sick dog and asks what symptoms the owner has observed in order to be able to diagnose the illness. Only then can he or she decide on an effective therapy, or on which diagnostic tests may be of value to arrive at the correct diagnosis.

Organization of the Section Describing Diseases

The diseases described in the following pages are divided into seven sections (on right). At the beginning of each section, the part of the body affected is shown in a schematized picture of a dog.

The descriptions of diseases follow this pattern:

Symptoms: First signs of the disease.

Causes: What triggers the disease.

Course: The course the disease may take.

● Treatment: What you can do yourself; what the veterinarian will prescribe; an arrow (➡)indicates when professional help is essential.

Follow-up care: What you should do after treatment is terminated.

Prevention: How the disease can be avoided.

■ Homeopathy: Suggestion of homeopathic remedies you can apply.

Susceptible breeds: Mention of breeds especially vulnerable to the disease.

Follow-up care, prevention, and susceptible breeds are not always applicable and therefore don't appear in every case.

Homeopathic treatments also are mentioned only if, in the author's opinion, they offer a good chance of success, particularly if used in conjunction with proper veterinary care.

The small picture on the right appears on every right-hand page and indicates which physical system is under discussion.

Homeopathy for Dogs

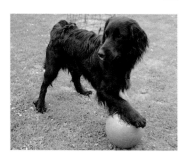

*W*hen a dog gets sick its owner is eager to try anything that promises to help his or her four-legged friend get well again. Often, too, the powerful drugs of orthodox medicine have undesirable side effects. That is why more and more people are exploring ways to treat their dogs with gentler yet effective methods. This is where homeopathy comes in. Homeopathic remedies assist the organism's efforts to heal itself but present no cause for worrying about harmful side effects. Homeopathy offers the animal lover a chance to supplement the care provided by the veterinarian.

Homeopathy Versus Veterinary Medicine

Since homeopathy is not being taught at veterinary schools, misunderstandings and confrontations between orthodox medicine (allopathy) and homeopathy unfortunately sometimes arise. Homeopathic treatment of a sick dog should not be undertaken in opposition to traditional veterinary medicine but rather in combination with and as a complement to it.

Homeopathy as a last resort? Sometimes when a very sick dog fails to respond to any of the allopathic methods tried, the owner may decide to consult a homeopath as a last resort. But you can't expect miracles from homeopathy. Instead, homeopathy should be regarded as an integral part of veterinary medicine and used in support of the body's own self-healing powers.

Applying homeopathy: It takes great sensitivity and much experience to practice homeopathy. Homeopathic remedies and their dilutions are as complex and varied as the causes of disease and the differences between individual dogs. There is consequently room for experimentation to test which remedies work best for which disease and for which dog. The

great advantage of homeopathic remedies is that they have no or almost no negative side effects.

Limits of homeopathy: If homeopathic treatments fail to show visible results within a reasonable time, you should consult a veterinarian without further delay. In this case other methods of treatment are called for. Homeopathy has also reached its limits when a disease has progressed to the point of producing changes in the organs or when homeopathic remedies no longer suffice to regulate and restore the body's functioning. That is why I have worked by the following rules for the past fifteen years:
• What responds to allopathic medicine should be treated by that method.
• Where surgery is called for, it should be performed.
• But there are a number of diseases that should be treated homeopathically because the two methods of treatment complement each other rather than work against each other.

The recommendations for treatment given in the following chapters are based on these principles. They are meant as guidelines promising a relatively high chance of success. All homeopathic remedies suggested have been tested by me in many years of practice.

What Is Homeopathy?

The term derives from the Greek words *homoios* (like) and *pathos* (suffering). Samuel Hahnemann (1755–1843), a physician, was the founder of homeopathy. This school of medicine is based on the theory that diseases can be cured by administering dilutions of substances that, if ingested undiluted, produce effects similar to those produced by the disease.

The basic assumption of homeopathy is the idea that life, including the life of our beloved pets, should be seen holistically. A well-balanced diet and proper living conditions are the basic necessities of a healthy dog. The dog's organism constantly undergoes an alternation of stress (metabolic processes, environmental effects) and relief (kidneys, liver, gall bladder, and intestines remove poisons from the body). If this balance between stress and relief is upset, even if in initially minor ways, the animal is sick. This is when homeopathy should be applied.

The self-healing powers of the body are supported or restored by homeopathic remedies, which do not suppress the symptoms of the disease. This is especially important in the case of puppies since their immune system and their resistance still have to be developed and strengthened.

A fever is basically a "healthy" response that shows that the immune system of the body is intact. As long as the dog fights the fever, the self-healing processes can be assisted with homeopathic remedies. The following remedies have shown good results: *Echinacea angustifolia, Aconitum, belladonna, ferrum phosphoricum, Vincetoxicum*, and chamomile (for restless puppies).

A temporary worsening of symptoms may occur in response to homeopathic remedies. But this "crisis" is the first step toward improvement and healing. There is no need for antibiotics unless or until the pathogens become too numerous and the body is no longer able to fight them on its own. If no improvement is seen in 24 to 48 hours, your veterinarian must be consulted.

The "Principle of Similarity"

The method of treatment proposed by Samuel Hahnemann rests on the following principle: In the case of some illnesses, certain substances have a curative effect on the organism when given in highly diluted form. If these same substances were given undiluted, they would cause the very disease that is being treated. *Similia similibus curentur,* which means "like is cured by like."

The example of bee poison: If bee poison *(apisinum)* enters a dog's body undiluted through a bee sting, the organism's reaction can take many different forms; there can be redness and swelling at the sting site; inflammation of the general area and also of the eyes, the heart, or the kidneys; fever and alternating depression and restlessness. Homeopathically prepared bee poison is used for diseases with the above mentioned symptoms. The highly diluted poison represents no danger to the body but instead briefly and subliminally rallies the organism's resistance. Vaccinations

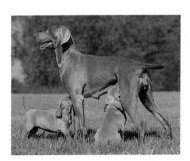

The smooth, shiny coat of this bitch attests to her good health.

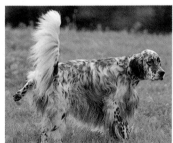

A male dog marks everything, even a tuft of grass.

work by the same principle. They, too, stimulate an immune reaction—though in this case a lasting one—against the injected pathogens.

Effects of Remedies
In the following paragraphs the effects of two homeopathic remedies for diarrhea are described. These examples illustrate how important it is to observe the sick animal very closely.

• *Arsenicum album*
A dog has licked up chemicals that contain white arsenic (providing an unintended experimental demonstration of the remedy's effects).

The following symptoms soon appear: rapidly increasing weakness, high fever, a facial expression of suffering, restlessness, fear, rapid weight loss, excessive thirst.

The stool is very runny, usually watery, and passage is preceded by colics. The dog's state deteriorates when the dog rests, that is, mostly at night, and when it is cold. The dog improves in a warm environment, whether damp or dry.

Treatment: If a dog suffering from diarrhea shows these specific symptoms, it should be treated with an appropriate dilution of *Arsenicum album.*

• *Nux vomica*
Another dog eats a bag of nutmeg in the kitchen. (*Nux moschata* is comparable to *Nux vomica* in its effects.)

The following symptoms are observed: Low fever, very little thirst even though the mouth is dry. There is bloating, and the stool, which is passed in small amounts and with great effort, is soft to runny. The dog responds to food with aversion. Its state of health declines if there are drafts and if the weather is wet and cold. Improvement is observed in a dry and warm environment.

Treatment: A dog suffering from diarrhea and displaying these symptoms should be treated homeopathically with *Nux vomica.*

Close observation and a careful diagnosis are necessary for successful homeopathic treatment. Consult with a homeopathic veterinarian. For addresses, see Homeopathic Veterinary Referral on page 126. The greater the similarity between the symptoms of the disease and the reaction to the remedy, the greater the likelihood that the treatment will accomplish a cure.

Manufacture of Remedies
Basic principles: Homeopathic remedies are derived from various natural sources. They may be of botanical or animal origin (such as bee and snake venom, deadly nightshade, monkshood) or chemical substances, such as sulfur, phosphorus, or mercury.

Manufacture: Homeopathic remedies are prepared in such a way that they can be used in various dilutions (potencies).

To dilute alcohol, one part "mother tincture" is added to 9 parts of the prescribed alcohol (a mixture of water and ethyl alcohol) and then vigorously mixed through repeated impact with a solid surface. This process adds further energy to the substance. At this first stage the remedy is said to be at first potency or at level D1 (D = decimal potency). The mother tincture is present in a ratio of 1 to 9. If one part of this D1 mixture is diluted with 9 parts alcohol, D2 is obtained. It contains the mother tincture in a ratio of 1 to 99. If one part D2 is mixed with 9 parts alcohol, we have D3, and so on.

As a general rule, the medium dilution ratios ranging from D6 to D10 should be used, for they are very unlikely to produce side effects. The low-numbered potencies D1 to D5 and the high-numbered ones above D10 should be used only if prescribed by an experienced homeopath.

In acute illnesses, the exact potency is of minor importance because any potency tends to help. Chronic illnesses call for higher-numbered potencies.

Availability: You can buy homeopathic remedies ready to use at pharmacies.

How to Give the Remedies
Homeopathic remedies are prepared in different forms.

Solid form: They are available as tablets, tiny little white pills (globuli), or powder (mixed with lactose) for oral consumption; as suppositories; or as salves that are rubbed into the skin.

Tablets work well for dogs because they can be mixed either whole or crushed into the food. Or one can crush a tablet, pick up the powder with a moistened finger tip, and dab it on the dog's tongue or gums.

Liquid form: Homeopathic remedies are also given as drops and as injections (administered by the vet). In liquid form, the remedies have a slight alcohol taste. They are convenient for sick dogs that are unable to eat solid food. The liquid is dribbled into the mouth with a little water (either directly or with a spoon or a syringe without the needle). The substance is absorbed directly by the mucous membranes of the mouth and goes to work quickly. With dogs that resist opening their mouth, the remedy can be dribbled or rubbed on the nose or paws, where the dog will lick it off.

How you administer the remedy depends on the animal, your own experience, and the illness that is being treated.

Storage
Homeopathic remedies are best kept in a cool, dry place. Close the containers tightly after use. Exposure to sunlight and strong-smelling substances can alter and even destroy homeopathic medicines. If stored properly, however, they keep for years.

Dosage

For an adult dog the dosage doesn't depend on the animal's size. A regular dose consists of
- 12 globuli;
- 1 tablet;
- ½ teaspoon powder; or
- 5 drops.

For acute illnesses homeopathic remedies can initially be given in quick succession, at a rate of one dose every 15 minutes to 1 hour for a full day or longer. As the animal's condition improves, the interval between doses is increased until the remedy is given only 3 or 4 times a day.

For chronic illnesses one dose is given once or twice a day.

Homeopathic treatment of specific illnesses is discussed in greater detail in the descriptions of diseases (pages 40–95), though only for conditions where this therapy makes sense. If no other dosage is mentioned, the one given above applies.

As a rule the medium potencies D6 to D10 should be used because they produce hardly any side effects (see above). More than one remedy can be given at once because different homeopathic medicines don't affect each other.

Disorders of the Digestive System

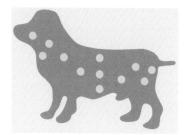

*T*he process of digestion starts when anticipation of food causes saliva to collect in the mouth. The food is swallowed in big chunks, and sometimes stones or even a small toy slides down the esophagus along with it. These objects can get stuck in the intestines and cause problems. The food is broken down in the stomach and the substances useful to the body absorbed in the small and large intestines. The indigestible parts are eliminated.

Tartar and Periodontosis

Symptoms: Bad breath, bloody saliva, problems chewing, brown and partially rock-hard coating on the teeth.

Causes: If the teeth don't get enough scrubbing because the food is too soft, tartar will form on them. Tartar consists of hardened salts from the saliva and of bits of food and bacteria present in the mouth.

Effects: Tartar causes inflammation of the gums (gingivitis), which leads to shrinking of the tissue is destroyed (periodontosis), the gums (periodontitis). In time the tissue is destroyed (periodontosis), the teeth become loose and fall out or have to be pulled if they become infected.

● Treatment
➡ The veterinarian can remove the tartar and extract loose or infected teeth. Dogs are usually anesthetized briefly for both cleaning and dental extraction. If a tooth was infected, antibiotic tablets have to be given for a week as well. Root canals, fillings, etc. also can be performed in canine dentistry.

Follow-up care: To assist healing and as a preventive measure, the teeth and the gums should be dabbed with a 1.5% hydrogen peroxide solution or a product containing chlorhexidin diacetate (available from the veterinarian or the drugstore). Apply it with a Q-tip.

Prevention: Let your dog chew regularly on a rawhide bone, a meat bone (veal or beef ball joint), or dried tripe for the mechanical friction and cleaning this provides for the teeth. You can also clean the dog's teeth. Pet stores and veterinarians sell tooth cleaning sets. Dogs that tend to develop tartar should be checked by the veterinarian every 3 to 4 months.

■ Homeopathy
For dosage, see page 39.

Mercurius solubilis Hahnemanni. Dab the gums and massage them with a salve (such as Traumeel). This also has an internal effect.
• If the gums tend to bleed: *Cinnamomum.*

Susceptible breeds: Particularly the toy versions of Yorkshire terriers, poodles, Chihuahuas, Pekingese, Shih Tzus, and Pomeranians tend to develop tartar and periodontosis. These dogs often

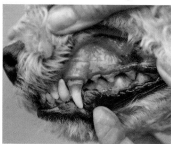

Periodontitis: Red and swollen gums recede from the teeth.

lose most of their teeth between the ages of 5 and 10 years if regular dental care is not provided.

Abscessed Tooth

Symptoms: Pain-sensitive swelling next to the maxillary bone just below the eye. This infection can break through the skin as a discharging sore. Often the eye is inflamed, too.

Cause: The dog has broken off a piece of a molar by biting down on a hard bone or a piece of wood or metal.

Effect: An infection enters the root canal through the break in the tooth.

● **Treatment**
➡ The veterinarian takes an X-ray to find out which root is affected. Depending on the recommendations of the veterinarian, the tooth may be extracted or root canal may be performed.

Follow-up care: To prevent the infection from spreading into the jaw, antibiotics in tablet form have to be given for at least a week.

Prevention: Train the dog not to chew on stones and metal.

■ **Homeopathy**
For dosage, see page 39.

Teeth that are infected over a period of time weaken the entire organism.

After the infected tooth is pulled, *Echinacea angustifolia, Echinacea purporea,* and

Aconitum should be given for about a week to clear the body of the poison.

Enlarged Gums and Tumors

Symptoms: Difficulties chewing, bad breath, sometimes bloody saliva.

Causes and effects: Growths on the gums most commonly take the following forms:
• Epulis: Hard, bony overgrowth of the gums that can become so big that the dog bites its own flesh and can no longer chew properly.
• Papilloma: Wart-like growths on the lips and the mucous membrane, usually in young dogs (caused by a virus).
• Malignant tumors: Growths in the mouth, on the jaw, and on the lips. Occur primarily in old dogs for reasons not yet understood. Often metastasize.

● **Treatment**
➡ Epulis and papilloma have to be removed by the veterinarian. These masses are generally not malignant but do sometimes recur in the same place. If a malignant growth has broken open, the veterinarian decides after a biopsy whether surgery makes sense or not. If the cancer has already spread to the nearby lymph nodes or the lungs, it is too late for surgery.

Follow-up care: To help the wound heal, irrigate it regularly with a camomile solution (use a syringe without the needle; available from the veterinarian or a drugstore).

Susceptible breeds: Epulis are relatively common in breeds

■ **Homeopathy for Enlarged Gums**
For epulida: Aurum metallicum, Thuja and *Calcium fluoratum* given together (contained in Galium-Heel, for example); preferably in increasing and then decreasing amounts, as follows:
1st day—1 drop 3 times
2nd day—2 drops 3 times
3rd day—3 drops 3 times
4th day—4 drops 3 times
5th day—5 drops 3 times
6th day—4 drops 3 times
7th day—3 drops 3 times
8th day—2 drops 3 times
9th day—1 drop 3 times

with short muzzles, especially boxers; watch out for malignant tumors in cockers, boxers, and pointers.

Cysts on the Salivary Glands

Symptoms: Blistery, fluid-filled swelling below the tongue (called "ranula" because it puffs up like the vocal pouch of a frog) or doughy, soft cyst on the neck; chewing problems; localized pain.

Causes: Blocking of the salivary ducts through thick saliva. The saliva collects in the tissue and forms a blister.

Effects: The blister gets inflamed and turns into an open abscess.

● **Treatment**
Ranula: A bulge under the tongue caused by accumulating secretion in a salivary gland.
➡ Has to be cut open by the vet. The incision usually heals quickly.
Cyst on the neck: Swelling caused by obstruction in salivary gland in the lower jaw.
➡ The cyst and the gland have to be removed surgically because otherwise cysts will continue to form.

Follow-up care: After the cyst has been removed, a drain must be installed so that the saliva will flow off until the stitches can be removed. (Put a protective bandage on the neck.)

Insect Bites

Symptoms: Sudden itching (the dog scratches its nose with its paws and rubs the muzzle against the ground), salivating, swelling, choking, vomiting, breathing difficulties.

Causes: Bee, wasp, or hornet stings in the mouth and throat.

Effects: Allergic reaction with serious swelling of the lips, tongue, or inside the mouth. The bigger the swelling in the mouth, the greater the danger of suffocation because of the narrowing of the air passages.

● **Treatment**
If the swelling is minor, dab the place with ice water or disinfecting alcohol (Isopropyl 50%, available at drugstores) until the swelling goes down.
➡ If the swelling is large and the dog salivates, vomits, and has trouble breathing, call the veterinarian immediately. He or she will give the dog antihistamines and/or cortisone (see Glossary, pages 114 and 115), to counteract the allergic reaction. If the throat swells shut, only a tracheotomy can save the animal.

Prevention: Break the dog of the habit of snapping at insects.

■ **Homeopathy**
Rub the stung area with salves containing *Apis, Echinacea angustifolia, Arnica, Calendula,* or *Hamamelis.*

Foreign Body in the Mouth or Throat

Symptoms: Drooling (sometimes with blood), swallowing difficulties, choking, vomiting, scratching at the mouth with the paws, swelling of the tongue. (It is important to note that drooling and difficulty in swallowing may be a sign of rabies. If the pet is not up to date in vaccines, the owner should only examine the oral cavity while wearing rubber gloves. If no foreign body is seen, a veterinarian should be consulted immediately.)

Causes: Splinters of bone or wood or fish bones stuck between the back teeth or

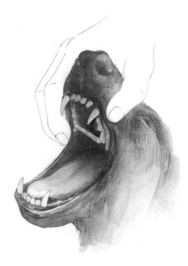

A splinter of wood has gotten stuck between the molars.

lodged in the back of the mouth or in the throat. Circular objects (ring-shaped cartilage, rubber bands, loops of thread) that have slipped around the tongue.

Effects: Jaws propped open by something stuck in the back of the mouth; acute urge to cough with efforts to spit up fish bone or splinter; later, inflammation and infection of the torn mucous membrane; and, eventually, formation of abscess in the throat. The tongue is swollen to huge size and may be bluish or partially necrotic because of lack of circulation.

● **Treatment**
➤ Professional help is needed. Examination and removal of the foreign body is generally possible only with the use of an anesthetic because dogs usually fight desperately any attempt to help them.

Follow-up care: Dab the injured mucous membranes with a 2 % silver nitrate or hydrogen peroxide solution or a chlorhexidine diacetate product (available from the veterinarian or a drugstore). Also give a decongestant twice a day if needed. If pus or an abscess forms, antibiotics are necessary.

Prevention: Don't give the dog chicken bones, large fish bones, or ring-shaped cartilage. When letting the dog play with a stick, make sure the ends are not split.

Important: Swelling of the tongue because of constriction

through a ring-shaped object is often mistaken for an insect bite. If the tongue is swollen very thick and has turned bluish, call the veterinarian immediately. The foreign object usually has to be located and removed under anesthesia.

Foreign Body in the Esophagus

Symptoms:
• If something has just gotten stuck: sudden restlessness, refusal to eat, salivating, choking up bits of food that may be bloody.
• If something has been lodged for some time: only intermittent choking; difficulty swallowing even liquids and mushy foods; drooling; swallowing the wrong way; sometimes coughing.

Causes: Foreign bodies, such as pieces of bone that are too large or pointed and fish hooks that have gotten stuck in the throat and block passage partially or completely.

Effects: A dog can get dehydrated because it keeps throwing up fluid. If the object stays stuck for some time, it causes inflammation. The dog loses weight because it can swallow only a small amount of food; it becomes increasingly apathetic as the infection spreads. This can go on for weeks.

If the foreign object does not block passage completely, the acute symptoms quickly sub-

side so that the dog owner no longer notices them. The chronic condition is then often misinterpreted and treated incorrectly.

● **Treatment**
➤ Professional help is required. A radiograph or fluoroscopy (see Glossary, page 116) is necessary to determine what exactly the foreign object is. It is then usually extracted from the throat or even the stomach with a probe while the dog is under anesthesia. Bones that are digestible can sometimes be pushed down into the stomach. Foreign bodies that were ingested some time ago and have caused chronic infection have to be surgically removed. Recovery depends on how far the infection has already spread (see Pneumonia and Pleurisy, pages 56 and 57).

Follow-up care: Intravenous therapy (see Glossary, page 117); in case of infected wounds in the throat, antibiotics. Liquid or soft food for 1 to 2 weeks.

Prevention: Don't let your dog play with pointed objects and don't give it large vertebrae to chew on. Exercise caution in your selection of toys for your pet.

■ **Homeopathy**
For dosage, see page 39.
Follow-up care: Pulsatilla, Nux vomica, Argentum nitricum.

Gastritis

Symptoms: Sudden vomiting (sometimes bloody), audible stomach rumbling, pain in the abdomen, increased thirst, vomiting after drinking water, dazed state, dehydration (see Glossary, page 116).

Causes: Spoiled food or food causing allergies, foreign body in the stomach, roundworms, poisoning, medications the animal doesn't tolerate, gastric ulcers. Infectious diseases like distemper and leptospirosis (see page 98 and 99) as well as chronic disorders of the liver and kidneys can also give rise to gastritis. A narrowing of the passage from the stomach to the intestine can also cause recurrent vomiting.

Effects: Frequent vomiting causes an acid-base imbalance in the body that may result in even more nausea and subsequent vomiting. If this condition continues for some time, a chronic gastritis (stomach inflamation) will occur.

● Treatment

If a dog vomits occasionally, all that is usually necessary is to withhold food for a day and then put the dog on a gastrointestinal diet (see page 24) for 1 to 3 days. If there is no improvement, take the animal to the vet.
➡ If vomiting persists and especially if it occurs spontaneously shortly after drinking, take the

dog to the veterinarian because there are a number of possible causes that require different treatment. Only the veterinarian can diagnose the problem accurately. He or she can control vomiting and prevent dehydration with intravenous therapy with saline and electrolyte solutions and by giving drugs that relieve cramping and the urge to vomit. There are also drugs that protect the stomach lining and substances, like baking soda, that neutralize the acid. In chronic gastritis, antacids (see Glossary, page 114), which inhibit the production of gastric acid, are effective.

Follow-up care: Gastrointestinal diet (see page 24) given in 3 to 4 small daily portions.

Prevention: Never serve food too hot or too cold. To prevent acidification of the stomach give the dog a small snack before going to bed. Never give medications on an empty stomach.

Stomach Ulcers and Tumors

Symptoms: Chronic vomiting (sometimes with bits of curdled blood), pain in the abdomen (especially shortly after meals), irregular appetite, dark to black feces (digested blood).

Causes: Ulcers are caused by overproduction of gastric acid, for example during chronic gastritis and some bacteria. The

■ Homeopathy for Gastritis

For dosage, see page 39.

Dogs are by nature carrion eaters. This is why their stomach lining produces a lot of gastric acid, which kills the bacteria in rotting food. If too much gastric acid is produced, which happens primarily if the stomach is empty, the dog wants to vomit and eats grass or swallows other things that may get stuck in the intestines.
• Give *Argentum nitricum, Acidum arsenicum, Nux vomica, Carbo vegetabilis.*
➡ In cases of frequent vomiting and especially if there is blood in the vomit, see the veterinarian.

cause of tumors is still unclear, but chronic inflammations seem to predispose to tumors.

Effects: Anemia as a result of steady loss of blood. Stomach bleeding, weight loss, perforated ulcer leading to acute peritonitis (see page 51).

● **Treatment**
➡ Professional help is required.

Diagnosis through radiography or endoscopy (see Glossary, page 116), or exploratory surgery may be required. Stomach tumors are difficult to diagnose because they are usually lodged deep in the stomach wall and alter the lining only minimally. The veterinarian generally prescribes a gastrointestinal diet (see page 24) and drugs. Sometimes surgery is required.

Follow-up care: See Gastritis, page 44. After surgery, intravenous feeding is usually required because no liquids can be given for 2 days and no solid food for 3 days.

Prevention: Treat chronic gastritis promptly and continue treatment long enough (a dog with a sensitive stomach may require special care for the rest of its life). Drugs that inhibit the production of gastric acid can prevent ulcers if given on a permanent basis.

Gastric Torsion

Symptoms: Sudden bloating of the stomach, often following a big evening meal. Restlessness, retching, salivating, vain attempts to vomit. Breathing difficulties.

Cause: If the dog has overeaten and there isn't enough gastric acid in the stomach to digest the food, the stomach empties too slowly. The food begins to ferment and produces increased gas that bloats the stomach and pulls it upward. At the same time the part of the stomach with food in it drops down, which causes a twist of the stomach around the vertical axis.

Effects: Closing of the esophagus and the duodenum. Further production of gas. Blood vessels are pinched and blood supply interrupted, which leads to weakened circulation, staggering, collapse, and death within a few hours.

● **Treatment**
➡ Acute emergency. Rush the dog to the veterinarian at the first sign. Generally only surgery can help to empty the stomach and unwind the twist. To prevent renewed twisting, the stomach is sewn to the abdominal wall.

Follow-up care: Intravenous feeding for 2 to 3 days after surgery. After that, put the dog on a gastrointestinal diet (see page 24) for 1 to 2 weeks. Antibiotics are given to prevent infection.

Prevention: Serve only small feedings, especially in the evening. Watch to make sure the dog is not rolling on its back immediately after eating.

■ **Homeopathy**
See Gastritis, page 44.

Susceptible breeds: Twisted stomach occurs primarily in large dogs, such as Great Danes, Saint Bernards, and German shepherds. It is rare in small dogs.

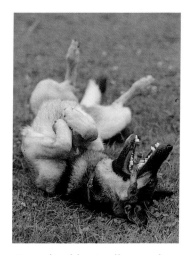

Dogs should not roll around immediately after eating; this can bring on a case of torsion.

Intestinal Obstruction (Blocked Bowel)

Symptoms: Lack of appetite, vomiting even after drinking water, no passage of stool, thick mucus in the rectum (it sticks to the thermometer when the rectal temperature is taken), apathy, abdominal pain.

Causes: Ingestion of a foreign body that is small enough to have passed through and out of the stomach but has gotten stuck in the small intestine; intussusception (the slipping of a length of intestine into the adjacent portion) or knotting of the intestines; in some dogs pinching of the intestine caused by a hernia (see page 49). Poisoning and infections can also result in paralysis of the intestines, which causes blockage of the ileum.

Effects: Foreign body stuck in the bowels can penetrate through the intestinal wall and cause acute peritonitis (see page 51) and eventually death.

● **Treatment**
➡ Rush the dog to the veterinarian; any delay may cost the dog's life. Radiology makes possible a precise diagnosis. Surgery is almost always necessary.
Follow-up care: After surgery, water is withheld for 1 day and food for 2 days while the dog is fed intravenously. Antibiotics are given for 1 week to prevent peritonitis.

Acute Enteritis

Symptoms: Diarrhea with soft to watery, sometimes bloody stool, usually accompanied by vomiting; general weakness; growling stomach; dehydration (see Glossary, page 116); sometimes a high fever.

Causes: Viral infections such as parvovirus disease or bacterical infections such as salmonellosis (see pages 99–100). Infection with coccidia (see page 102).

Effects: Viral infections are often fatal for puppies up to 6 months old.

● **Treatment**
➡ Consult the veterinarian. Take a stool sample along because the pathogens may be present in the feces. Sometimes they can be determined through blood tests. Depending on the nature of the pathogen different drugs are prescribed. Fluids are given intravenously. Also important are a diet for gastrointestinal problems (see page 24), sweetened black tea, and drugs to relax cramping of the intestines and to protect the mucous lining (carbonic acid and tannic acid tablets and kaolin, pectin, or bismuth subsulphate).

Follow-up care: Intensive care, usually in an animal clinic, may be necessary for several days or weeks.

Prevention: Don't let the dog eat indiscriminately; make sure it gets a well-balanced diet. Vaccinations and dewormings at the proper times are important, especially for puppies (see Vaccination Schedule, page 20).

■ **Homeopathy**
For dosage, see page 39.
• To neutralize toxic gases and materials: *Carbo vegetabilis.*
• For cramps and the urge to defecate, especially when it's cold: *Nux vomica.*
• For very runny diarrhea, especially at night: *Veratrum.*

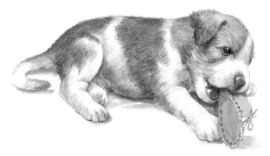

Puppies eat all kinds of things while playing. Sometimes, intestinal obstruction can result. A toy made of rawhide makes a good plaything.

• For colic before diarrhea and exhaustion set in: *Arsenicum album* (exposure to warmth often brings relief).

Chronic Enteritis

Symptoms: Occasional vomiting; lack of appetite or, sometimes, voracious eating; weight loss; dull, ragged coat; alternating consistency of feces; bloating; occasionally worms and sometimes blood in the stool.

Causes and Effects:
• Intestinal parasites (coccidia, *Giardia,* hookworms, whipworms, roundworms, or tapeworms; see pages 101 and 102) deprive the dog's body of too many nutrients, leading to weight loss.
• Bacteria overwhelm the beneficial intestinal flora and interfere with normal digestion.
• Foreign bodies that get hung up in the small intestine without completely blocking it (such as buttons and pieces of bone) impede the passage of food and lead to digestive problems.
• Chronic underactivity of the pancreas or chronic liver damage result in incomplete digestion of the food eaten. The dog loses weight in spite of voracious appetite.

● **Treatment**
➡ Visit the veterinarian and take along a stool sample. Examination of the stool sample may reveal the presence of parasites or bacteria, and proper treatment can bring relief. If there is a foreign body, surgery is usually necessary. For treatment of an underactive pancreas or chronic kidney or liver disease, see pages 51, 66, and 50, respectively.

Follow-up care: Antibiotics for at least 1 week. Make sure the dog gets a strict gastrointestinal diet (page 24).

Prevention: Regular deworming. This is as important as regular vaccinations (see Vaccination Schedule, page 20).

■ **Homeopathy**
See Acute Enteritis, page 46.

Chronic Colitis

Symptoms: Variable consistency of the stool. Obvious attempts to defecate during which the dog moves forward in a crouching position. Feces covered with a slimy film that sometimes envelops them almost like a skin. Stool is passed in small amounts, frequently, sometimes uncontrolled, and often mixed with blood (fresh, undigested red blood from the rectum).

Causes: Bacterial infection of the mucous lining in the colon, usually accompanied by ulceration. Restlessness, nervousness, and anxiety speed up the passage of digested matter through the colon, resulting in runny mucus-laden stool.

Effects: Increased secretion of mucus causes damage in the deeper layers of the colon's lining, which leads to larger and larger ulcers.

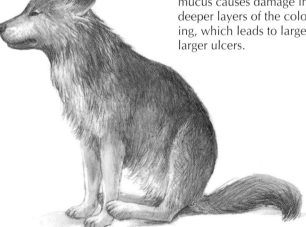

Dogs that drag their rears along the ground ("scooting") may have dirty and sticky anuses, worms, or inflamed anal sacs.

● **Treatment**

If chronic colitis is caused by nervousness, tranquilizers are often effective. If caused by bacteria, antibiotics are prescribed.

Only a veterinarian can correctly diagnose what is causing ulceration in the colon. The basis of treatment is a strict gastrointestinal diet (see page 24) plus black tea, tablets of activated charcoal, and medications containing tannic acid, which help produce more solid feces. In addition, cramp- and pain-relieving drugs are given. If there are ulcers, cortisone (see Glossary, page 115) may be prescribed as well.

Follow-up care: Therapy has to be continued for several weeks and sometimes for months. Often the dog has to stay on a special diet for life.

■ **Homeopathy**

For dosage, see page 39.

Podophyllum, Ignatia, Mercurius sublimatus corrosivus, graphites, Aloe, Veratrum. Don't feed the dog organ meats.

Susceptible breeds: Boxers, Dobermans, German shepherds, and Irish setters tend to have nervous diarrhea and chronic colitis. Boxers are subject to a hereditary form of ulcerative colitis.

Fecal Impaction

Symptoms: Constant urge to defecate without result. Usually the dog passes partially bloody mucus. Cries of pain, licking of the anus; and, if condition persists, vomiting and dehydration.

Causes: Ingestion of too many bones, such as pork ribs, oxtail, or poultry bones, can lead to rock-hard feces in the rectum and to constipation. In old male dogs fecal impaction is sometimes caused by an enlarged prostate that presses on the colon (see Hernia, page 49). Poultry bones, especially chips of the long hollow bones, sometimes get lodged sideways in the rectum so that stool cannot be passed because of the pain it causes. As mentioned, these bones should never be offered to dogs.

Effects: Poisoning of the body through metabolic by-products; peritonitis; abscesses in the anus.

● **Treatment**

➡ Take a dog with fecal impaction to your veterinarian without delay. X-rays can determine how serious the situation is. Often, enemas can bring relief. Occasionally the animal has to be anesthestized and the bone-containing feces broken up and removed. Bone splinters lodged in the intestine have to be extracted one by one.

Follow-up care: Add a mild laxative prescribed by your veterinarian to the regular food for a few days to keep the stool soft. Ointments for hemorrhoid relief help reduce inflammation of the anal region.

Prevention: Always feed the dog a well-balanced diet. Avoid giving the dog any bone that it can chew up and swallow.

■ **Homeopathy**

For dosage, see page 39.

• For animals that are sensitive to the cold: *Natrium chloratum.*
• In case of cramps: *Atropinum.*

Hernia

Symptoms: Severe pain, restlessness, a bulge at the navel (umbilical hernia), in the groin (inguinal hernia), or in the rectal area between the anus and the genitals (perineal hernia).

Causes: A hernia is a sacklike protrusion of the peritoneum through an opening in the abdominal wall. Parts of the intestine or of another abdominal organ push through the hole and lie just under the skin. Hernias occur if muscles are suddenly overstrained or torn, as may happen in an accident, or because of increased pressure in the abdominal cavity during pregnancy.

• Since the navel and the inguinal canal are gaps in the abdominal wall that are present

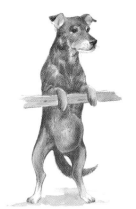

To detect hernias have it stand up on its hind legs. In that position a bulge is visible.

from birth, hernias can occur in newborn puppies.

• Hernias in the prostate area happen primarily to old males that are constipated and strain constantly because the prostate gland is enlarged (see Fecal Impaction, page 48).

Effects: Minor hernias in which no intestines protrude cause no discomfort. Large ones interfere with intestinal motility. If parts of the intestine are pinched, this can lead to intestinal obstruction and gangrene (see page 46).

● **Treatment**

➡ A strangulated hernia (where blood supply to tissue is cut off) represents an emergency, and professional help must be sought immediately. All other hernias should at some point be operated on if they are large or cause discomfort.

Follow-up care: A mild laxative prescribed by your veterinarian should be added to the food for a few days to help keep the stool soft. It makes sense to operate on a hernia in the prostate area only if the dog is neutered at the same time, so that the prostate gland will shrink.

Prevention: As a general rule, have a hernia operated on in good time, before it becomes strangulated. Umbilical hernias should, if possible, be surgically corrected while the puppy is young.

Anal Tumors and Anal Sac Abscesses

Symptoms: Pustules around the anus, sometimes breaking open with blood and pus; "scooting" (see Glossary, page 118); constant licking of the anal area; foul to sour smell.

Causes and Effects:

• The openings of the anal sacs or glands can become plugged if the secretion (see Glossary, page 118) becomes viscid. This causes impaction of the glands. If bacteria are present, inflammation and abscessation of the gland will occur.

• Anal tumors occur primarily in old male dogs and are generally not malignant. Occasionally they break through the skin, forming a bleeding, crater-like wound.

● **Treatment**

➡ Take the dog to the veterinarian. Inflamed anal glands, especially in the form of abscesses, subside relatively quickly if incised and irrigated with a diluted antiseptic solution and if antibiotics are given. If the inflammation recurs, the glands should be surgically removed.

Anal tumors are usually harmless, but if they open up and bleed, they should be surgically removed. They can, however, grow back. Some are malignant and can be life threatening.

Follow-up care: A hemorrhoid ointment applied to the area around the anus relieves itching. The dog should be given antibiotics for a week after an abscess breaks open or is treated surgically.

Prevention: Hormone treatments or neutering can significantly lower the recurrence of tumors.

■ **Homeopathy**

For dosage, see page 39.

If the skin of the anal region and lips is dry and cracked: *Paeonia afficinalis, Acidum nitricum.*

Liver Disease

In dogs, as in man, the liver is the prime organ involved in the metabolic process. It transforms carbohydrates, proteins, and fats into the substances the organism needs to function. It is therefore not surprising that a malfunctioning liver has major consequences.

Liver disease manifests itself in the following general symptoms: Tiredness; poor appetite; weight loss; sometimes vomiting; diarrhea with light colored stool; increased thirst; spontaneous bleeding; anemia; jaundice; dark, brownish urine; complete apathy; abnormal movement; staggering; epileptic seizures; coma.

Serious symptoms to watch out for: Jaundice, enlarged liver (area in the upper abdomen that is hard to the touch and painful), pale yellowish stool, dark brown urine, fluid in the abdomen (swollen, wobbly belly). These symptoms are caused by one of two diseases that take different courses, namely, acute and chronic hepatitis.

Tumors of the liver are relatively rare, but when they occur they are usually malignant. They are generally the result of metastasis (see Glossary, page 118) associated with cancer of the spleen or pancreas or with leukemia (see page 62).

Acute Hepatitis

Causes: Infectious diseases (see pages 98–101) caused by viruses, bacteria, or parasites in the blood. Poisoning through medications, insecticides, or other toxic substances.

● **Treatment**
➡ Rush the animal to the veterinarian because its life may be in danger. The first emergency measure is intravenous fluid therapy. Then appropriate drugs, such as antibiotics, are administered to fight the disease that has caused hepatitis. If a dog survives the acute phase it can—as in the case of a chronic liver disease—quite often be helped. The liver is often capable of recovering even from very serious disease if properly treated.

■ **Homeopathy for Liver Disease**

For dosage, see page 39.
• If lack of appetite, bloating, ascites: *Lycopodium.*
• If accumulation of bile (jaundice): *Taraxacum, Carduus marianus, Vincetoxicum, Chelidonium.*
• If vomiting bile: *Leptandra.*
• If major weight loss: *China.*
Don't use drops because these contain alcohol.

Chronic Hepatitis

Causes: Cortisone level too high in the blood because of overactive adrenal glands (see page 86) or because of prolonged, high-dosage cortisone therapy; improper fat metabolism brought on by a diet high in fat, obesity, or diabetes; chronic infections; poisoning with heavy metals or insecticides; chronic vascular congestion of the liver.

Effects: Fat in the liver and cirrhosis of the liver.

● **Treatment**
➡ Professional help is required. Blood tests (to check liver function and presence of antibodies) or a biopsy (see Glossary, page 114) of liver tissue are used to arrive at a precise diagnosis.

Treatment consists of fighting the underlying disease and in adhering to a strict liver diet (see page 24). Usually antibiotics have to be administered initially to prevent further infections. Low doses of cortisone (see Glossary, page 115) can sometimes reduce cirrhosis of the liver.

Follow-up care: Antibiotics for 1 to 2 weeks. Strict liver diet. Regular checks of liver function (at first weekly, later once a month).

Pancreatic Insufficiency

The pancreas produces both the enzymes that digest the food in the intestines and insulin, which regulates the blood sugar level. Impaired functioning of the pancreas without inflammation eventually leads to diabetes (see page 87). Inflammation and the resulting shrinking of the organ affects primarily the effectiveness of digestion (malabsorption syndrome). Acute inflammation of the pancreas is not uncommon in obese dogs, especially after a high fat meal. It may result in serious illness or in fatal peritonitis.

Symptoms: In chronic pancreatic malfunction or insufficiency (atrophy of the pancreas): Weight loss in spite of normal or voracious appetite; stool varies in consistency, is ochre colored, and glistens as though greased; constant digestive problems with occasional vomiting; bloating; diarrhea.

Causes and effects: The atrophying of the digestive part of the pancreas results in decreased production of gastric juices (enzymes) and consequently to chronic digestive problems.

● **Treatment**
➡ Professional help is required. Analysis of stool samples reveals if there is a lack of digestive enzymes. After inflammation—if present—has been resolved, enzymatic agents for the digestion and a diet high in easily digestible proteins and carbohydrates but low in fat is prescribed.

Follow-up care: Substitutes for the enzymes produced by the pancreas must be supplied in the food, and a strict pancreatic diet (see page 25) has to be maintained for the rest of the dog's life. Give the food in 3 to 4 daily portions. In spite of good care, digestive problems may recur, which will, depending on the symptoms, have to be treated like chronic enteritis (see page 47).

■ **Homeopathy**
For dosage, see page 39.
   To assist recovery:
• if there is recurrent vomiting and white to grayish stool: *Acidum phosphoricum;*
• if there is diarrhea: *Arsenicum album.*
   Don't use drops; they contain alcohol.

Susceptible breeds: German shepherds have a heritable tendency to develop chronic atrophy of the pancreas at 1½ to 2 years of age. Animals suffering from the disease should not be bred.

Peritonitis

Symptoms: Weakness, high fever, vomiting, rapid breathing, racing pulse, arched back, severe pain in the abdomen, movements and lying down slowly and cautiously because the belly hurts so much.

Causes: Infection in the peritoneal cavity because a foreign body has pierced the intestine or because of external injury; injuries of the stomach, intestines, or bladder caused by an accident; uterine infection (pyometra) with the abscess breaking open or an open abscess on the prostate; acute inflammation of the pancreas.

Effects: If not treated, peritonitis leads to death within a few days.

● **Treatment**
➡ Professional help is required. If the animal's general health is poor, intravenous fluid therapy (see Glossary, page 117) is necessary. High doses of antibiotics and anti-inflammatory analgesics help combat acute symptoms. After these initial emergency measures, it is crucial to treat the underlying disease. To accomplish this, surgical opening, drainage, and irrigation of the peritoneal cavity is generally required.

Follow-up care: Generally, intravenous fluid therapy and irrigation drainage of the peritoneal cavity are necessary for 3 to 4 days. Antibiotics are given for 1 to 2 weeks.

Disorders of the Respiratory and Circulatory Systems

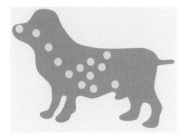

Dogs depend on air for life just as humans do. The air is inhaled through the nose and mouth and travels through the trachea to the lungs, where it supplies the blood with oxygen. The blood flows to the heart and is pumped from there through the aorta and the arteries to all parts of the body. The oxygen-depleted blood then returns through the veins to the heart and then the lungs, where it gives off carbon dioxide and absorbs new oxygen.

Wounds on the Front of the Nose

The skin on the nose and around the nostrils generally includes dark pigments, is covered with a thin layer of keratinous cells, and is smooth and usually moist. However, a dry, hot nose doesn't necessarily signal illness. Instead, a dry nose or cracks in the skin are often a hereditary trait. Dogs that try to bury bones or other food on a rough wooden floor or a rug often have scabs and abrasions on the nose. A chronic distemper infection sometimes also leads to a horn-like hard scabbing of the nose skin. Various autoimmune disorders (see pages 84 and 95) can be accompanied by weeping sores around the nostrils.

Treatment: Rub some baby or other massage oil onto the nose skin to prevent drying out. For wounds and scabs, medication containing oily antibiotics and cortisone, dispensed by the veterinarian, may be used.

Rhinitis

Symptoms: Noisy breathing; sneezing; watery, purulent mucus, and sometimes bloody discharge from the nose; pus and scabs on the sides of the nose; if nose is plugged up, noisy breathing through the mouth; pumping exhalation through the nose.

Causes: Inflammation of the mucous membranes usually caused by a virus. Often leads to purulent discharge from the nose if accompanied by a bacterial infection. Rhinitis can also be a symptom of distemper or kennel cough (see pages 98 and 100). If the discharge is mostly from one nostril, it is usually caused by a foreign object or a tumor.

Effects: Chronic rhinitis, which frequently leads to a fungus infection. This can result in the destruction of nasal cartilage.

● Treatment

In case of a simple cold, clean the nostrils 3 times a day with some cotton moistened with lukewarm camomile tincture. Inhalation (see Glossary, page 117) of vapors from eucalyptus oil may provide some relief and comfort.

➡ In case of pus-producing rhinitis, visit the veterinarian. Irrigation of the deeper-lying regions of the nose and examination to see if a foreign body is in the nose have to be performed under anesthesia.

Anesthesia is also necessary for taking X-rays if there is a suspicion of tumors or of inflammation in the sinus cavities. Decongestant nose drops have a healing effect, and antibiotics are given if there is a severe infection and high fever. Fungus infections can usually be cured only through a surgical reaming of the nasal cavities. There is a 70% chance that tumors in the nose are malignant, and many of them are inoperable.

Note: Nosebleeds can be caused by foreign bodies, tumors, fungus induced rhinitis, abscessed teeth, and broken blood vessels. But they can also be a symptom of abnormal blood clotting, poisoning, severe liver disease, or leukemia. As a first-aid measure, apply ice water and plug the affected nostril. Then rush the animal to the veterinarian.

Follow-up care: Especially in the case of fungal infections, treatment with antimycotics (see Glossary, page 114) often has to be continued for weeks or months.

Prevention: Clean the front of the nose every morning.

■ Homeopathy
For dosage, see page 39.
Euphorbium, Mercurius bijodatus.
• In case of mucus discharge: *Pulsatilla.*
• In case of bleeding: *Cinnamomum.*

Susceptible breeds: Short-nosed, small breeds, such as pugs, Pekingese, French bulldogs, and Boston terriers. If the wings of the nose are too wide, one or both nostrils collapse when the dog inhales, shutting off the air. Sometimes this birth defect has to be surgically corrected.

Sore Throat, Tonsillitis, and Laryngitis

Symptoms: Rattling breath and snoring, especially if the dog is excited or hot; also heavy panting, choking fits, swallowing difficulties, frequent empty swallowing with outstretched neck, expectorant cough sometimes combined with vomiting, hoarse barking.

Causes: In short-nosed breeds, the oral cavity may be too narrow, which tends to encourage infection; colds; insect bites (see page 42); foreign body in the throat; edema of the larynx; paralysis of the vocal cords; tumors in the oral cavity.

Effects: Chronic inflammation of the throat and tonsils can lead to lung disease and disorders of the gastrointestinal tract. Chronic conditions can also be caused by tumors and other growths.

● Treatment
You can recognize laryngitis and pharyngitis by the enlarged, visible tonsils and by the reddened,

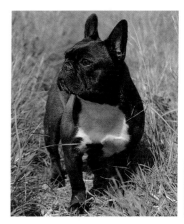

Dogs with short noses are subject to disorders of the mouth and throat.

mucus-covered throat. In mild cases, keeping the dog warm by putting a scarf around its neck (see drawing, page 54) and giving it soft, warmed-up food help.
➡ If there is no improvement, take the dog to the veterinarian. He or she may paint the throat with a mucus-dissolving drug (containing codeine) that relieves the urge to cough. Sulfa drugs and antibiotics (see Glossary, pages 119 and 114) keep serious, purulent infections from becoming chronic. Tonsillectomy is rarely necessary. Foreign bodies in the throat (fish or other bones, wood splinters, fish hooks) have to be removed under anesthesia. Edema and cramping of the larynx are treated with antihistamines and antispasmodic drugs. Tumors, paralysis of the vocal cords, and an enlarged

soft palate usually have to be surgically treaeted.

Follow-up care: Give the dog decongestants and antibiotics for at least 1 week and keep it warm.

Prevention: Make sure nothing the dog eats and drinks is too hot or too cold.

■ Homeopathy
For dosage, see page 39.
• For tonsilitis: *Mercurius solubilis, Lachesis, belladonna, Echinacea angustifolia.*
• For high fever, swallowing difficulties, and gnashing of teeth: *Phytolacca.*
• For laryngitis and hoarse barking: *Phosphorus.*
• For laryngitis with a barking cough and much mucus: *Drosera.*

Susceptible breeds: Short-nosed breeds, such as Pekingese, pugs, Boston terriers, French bulldogs, and boxers, suffer from these problems more than other dogs because of their narrow mouths. Excitement, heat, minor inflamed swellings, and mucus in the throat all can cause severe breathing difficulties. In most cases surgical correction of the soft palate is necessary to prevent recurring problems.

Wearing a warm scarf often helps a sore throat feel better.

Inflammation of the Windpipe (Tracheitis)

Symptoms: Fits of dry, hacking coughing often brought on by being pulled on the leash, by fresh air, or by swallowing the wrong way when drinking. Breathing difficulties and rattling noises especially during inhaling.

Causes: Constriction or collapse of the windpipe caused by tumors, swelling of lymph nodes, the formation of abscesses because of a foreign body in the throat, and also enlargement of the heart.

Effects: Constriction or collapse of the trachea interferes with breathing, causing endless coughing fits.

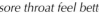

● Treatment
➡ Take the dog to the veterinarian. For a precise diagnosis of tracheitis, X-rays are necessary and usually tracheoscopy as well. Both have to be done under anesthesia. Treat with expectorant drugs, antibiotics, and inhalations (see Glossary, page 117). If the trachea is constricted, the causative agent, such as a tumor or foreign body, has to be surgically removed if possible.

Follow-up care: Expectorants, antibiotics, antispasmodics, and inhalation therapy have to be continued for 1 to 2 weeks.

Prevention: If you put a harness (available at pet stores) on your dog for walking, you won't have to pull on the dog's collar. Dogs with a congenitally flattened windpipe should not be bred.

Susceptible breeds: Toy versions of Yorkshire terriers, poodles, Pomeranians, and Shih Tzus tend to have a congenitally flattened windpipe. An overly narrow windpipe is a birth defect also found in English bulldogs, mastiffs, and related breeds.

■ Homeopathy
See Bronchitis, page 55.

Bronchitis, Foreign Bodies in the Bronchi

Symptoms: Long fits of a deep, wet, often whistling cough; breathing difficulties especially in exhaling; slow exhaling accompanied by whistling noises.

Causes: Infection involving various viruses (see Kennel Cough, page 100), bacteria, some rare parasites; almost always accompanied by tracheobronchitis. Harmful, irritating environmental substances, allergic reaction to insect bites, hypersensitivity to drugs; inhaling of foreign bodies (grasses, grains, small stones, wood chips, dust).

Effects: Foreign bodies that are not coughed up can lead, after a few days or weeks, to pneumonia (see page 56). Allergic bronchitis may bring on asthma.

● Treatment

In the early stages, warmth, rubbing in and compresses of alcohol and camphor salves, perhaps combined with inhalations (see Glossary, page 117) help.
➡ If there is a fever, take the dog to the veterinarian. Medications that loosen the mucus and open up the bronchi are prescribed, and, if the urge to cough is very strong, codeine or even tranquilizers. If the bronchi are

dilated (bronchiectasis), antibiotics and sulfa drugs are usually necessary, too. If parasites are involved, these are treated with the appropriate drugs. Bronchitis caused by allergies—which occur in dogs with increasing frequency because of growing air pollution—is treated with cortisone and/or antihistamines. Foreign bodies are removed either through bronchoscopy or endoscopy (see Glossary, page 116) or, if they are infected or impacted, through surgery.

Follow-up care: Antibiotics for 1 to 2 weeks; expectorant drugs until the symptoms recede, especially if there is a tendency to develop chronic bronchitis. Bronchitis caused by allergy often requires lifelong low-dose cortisone treatments.

Prevention: Dry air aggravates the tendency to develop bronchitis. That is why it is important in centrally heated rooms to maintain adequate air humidity (50–60%). For dogs—as for people—tending to chronic bronchitis, inhalation of vapors and aerosols (see Glossary, page 114) is an optimal preventive measure (see drawing). Time spent in the bracing mountain or sea air also has a long-term prophylactic effect.

■ Homeopathy

For dosage, see page 39.

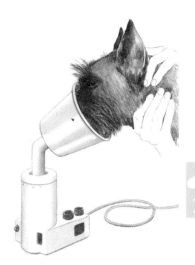

For inhalation treatments, hold the dog's nose into the mouthpiece of the inhalator with gentle pressure.

Tartarus stibiatus, Drosera, Hepatica triloba.
● For dry cough: *Naphtalium.*
● If coughing in the evening and at night: *Ipecacuanha.*
● For short, dry cough: *Arsenicum jodatum.*
● For a convulsive, asthma-like state: *Cuprum sulfuricum* (in the form of suppositories).
● If the mucus cannot be coughed up: *Coccus cacti.*

Pneumonia

Symptoms: Usually a high fever (up to 106°F or 41°C); apathy; wet, weak, and usually painful cough that can be set off by tapping the dog's chest; purulent discharge from the nose and mucopurulent conjunctivitis; labored breathing with shorter, more rapid breaths than usual.

Causes: An inflammation of the entire lungs that may follow a not completely healed bronchitis or be triggered by an infectious disease, such as distemper. Puppies are especially susceptible. Other possible causes are heart disease and congested lungs, allergies, injuries to the pectoral area, and foreign bodies that have caused infection (see Bronchitis, page 55). Severe pneumonia may result from getting food into the trachea when, for instance, the dog loses consciousness, is under anesthesia, or is being force fed, and from abnormal swallowing associated with diseases of the trachea.

Effects: Severe pneumonia that is already at an advanced stage leads to permanent lung damage and is often fatal.

● **Treatment**
➡ The veterinarian determines the severity and causative agent of the disease with the help of blood tests, cultures, and radiographs. The treatment is the same as for bronchitis.

Follow-up care: Depending on the causative agent, antibiotics and antimycotics (see Glossary, page 114) often have to be given over a period of weeks or months. A climate with contrasts in temperature as in the mountains and by the ocean also has a beneficial effect.

Prevention: To prevent pneumonia caused by swallowing the wrong way under anesthesia, don't give your dog anything to eat for 12 hours before anesthesia is administered.

■ **Homeopathy for Pneumonia**

For dosage, see page 39.

Since pneumonia is almost always accompanied by high fever, antibiotics are necessary. Homeopathic remedies are recommended only to assist healing and for the convalescent period.

To assist the healing process:
● When pneumonia first starts: *Aconitum.*
● For severe breathing difficulties, gasping, or whistling noises during inhalation, and especially if the cough is worse at night and the dog is unable to sleep lying down: *belladonna.*

During convalescence: *Drosera,* Phosphorus.

For strengthening the heart: *Crataegus.*

Pulmonary Edema

Symptoms: Shortness of breath, restlessness; dogs seek out cool places and fresh air; weak, wet cough; bubbly, white sputum; bluish mucous membranes. Dogs pant with exhaustion while standing or sitting. Irregular, fast pulse.

Causes: The most common cause is heart disease, in which the blood backs up in the lungs, resulting in an abnormal accumulation of fluid in the lung tissues. Other possible causes are poisoning and insect bites (see page 42).

Effects: If pulmonary edema is not treated, the dog may suffocate.

● **Treatment**
➡ Acute symptoms of pulmonary edema develop only gradually. Once the condition has been determined, the veterinarian provides increased oxygen supply; the dog is calmed possibly with sedatives. Drugs are given to reduce fluids in the body and the lungs and to open the bronchi. Mucus is sucked from the mouth and throat. Depending on the cause triggering the condition, other drugs may be necessary, such as cortisone, heart stimulants, and antidotes for poisons.

Follow-up care: Once the dog is past the critical phase, circulation has to be stabilized with heart medication and diuretics (sometimes for the rest of the dog's life).

Prevention: If a dog has heart disease, avoid excitement, exertion, obesity, and, especially, humid heat.

■ Homeopathy

For dosage, see page 39.

Apis, Crataegus, Kalium carbonicum.

Lung Cancer

Cancer very rarely starts in the lungs. In these rare cases, surgery offers some hope in the very early stages. Considerably more common are metastases (see Glossary, page 118) of other forms of cancer, such as breast and bone cancer. Tumors in the lungs can be detected with X-rays once they reach a certain size (about ¼ inch or 5 mm). Surgery is usually countereffective since it tends to accelerate metastasis. The best thing you can do is to make the remaining life of your dog as pleasant as possible and to call the veterinarian at the appropriate time to cut suffering short by putting the dog to sleep (see page 113).

Pleurisy and Effusions into the Thoracic Cavity

Symptoms: Weak, suppressed, painful cough; sometimes fever; accelerated breathing, often with noticeable movement of the abdominal wall; pumping breathing when standing or sitting still, restlessness until exhaustion sets in.

Causes: Bacterial, fungal and viral infections, tears in the trachea caused by a foreign body, or injury to the chest wall.

Effusions into the thoracic cavity are caused by fluid in the lungs (see page 56), as well as by injured blood vessels and tumors in the thoracic cavity.

Effects: The lungs can no longer expand because of fluid, and the dog suffocates.

● Treatment

➡ Rush the animal to the veterinarian, who will investigate with X-rays, blood tests, or by

drawing off a sample of the fluid. If there is a fever, this suggests infection, and the condition is treated with pain killers, cough suppressants with codeine, and antibiotics. In case of chronic infection, irrigation of the thoracic cavity with a sterile saline solution is helpful. If heart disease is involved, heart medication and diuretics are required. Surgery is sometimes effective against tumors or can repair tears in the lungs and damaged blood vessels.

Follow-up care: Antibiotics.

Prevention: Make sure bronchitis and pneumonia are completely healed.

■ Homeopathy

For dosage, see page 39.

Prolonged disease of the lungs and pleura strain the heart.

• To strengthen the heart: *Crataegus or Cactus.*

• Otherwise: *Bryonia alba, Lachesis,* phosphorus.

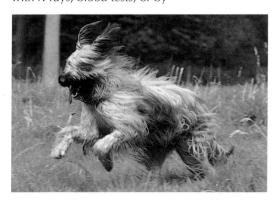

If a dog has heart problems (see page 39), it should not race around too wildly.

Air in the Pleural Cavity (Pneumothorax)

Symptoms: Pumping breathing, increased pulse rate, shortness of breath without audible breathing noises, bluish tongue and mucous membranes.

Causes: The impact of being hit by a car can cause small tears in the lung tissues through which air escapes into the pleural cavity. The lungs shrivel, which cuts down on the amount of air that can be inhaled.

Effects: The dog may suffocate.

● **Treatment**
See Emergency Measures, page 26, and Air in the Pleural Cavity, page 27. Then rush the dog to the veterinarian.
➡ X-rays show how much air is in the pleural cavity (pneumothorax). If the capacity of the lungs is reduced to less than one-third the normal volume, air has to be sucked out. Then the lungs can expand again.

Follow-up care: Provide fresh air, quiet, and warmth. If the air did not have to be drawn off, the body absorbs it within a day or two. If a fever develops in the process, antibiotics have to be given to prevent pleurisy.

Prevention: Keep dogs leashed when in traffic.

Defects and Tears in the Diaphragm

Symptoms: Pumping breathing, forced exhalation in which the abdominal wall is pressed in to make up for the defective diaphragm; shortness of breath, bluish mucous membranes; occasionally vomiting, belching up of air; if condition persists, emaciation and death.

Causes: Tears in the diaphragm can result from the impact and contusion sustained in an accident. Small defects can be present from birth and go undetected for years.

Effects: Migration of abdominal organs (stomach, intestines, spleen, liver) into the pleural thoracic cavity. This significantly interferes with breathing and can lead to suffocation.

● **Treatment**
➡ Rush the animal to the veterinarian. Radiographic studies using contrast media that register on film reveal the parts of the liver, stomach or intestines that have migrated into the thoracic cavity. Tears and defects in the diaphragm can be corrected only through surgery, during which the animal has to be on an artificial respirator because the thoracic cavity is open on the abdominal side until the defect is surgically repaired.

Follow-up care: Antibiotics given for 1 week prevent pleurisy from developing. The dog should stay at the animal clinic for 2 to 3 days where breathing and circulation can be monitored.

Chronic Valvular Heart Disease

Symptoms: Occasional coughing, weakness, especially after exertion and excitement; listlessness, primarily during hot, sticky weather; shortness of breath; increasing belly size; swelling (edema) of the legs, lower chest, and the abdomen; restlessness, especially at night; occasional fainting fits.

Causes: Chronic valvular heart disease develops with age (see also Congenital Heart Diseases, page 59), setting in at age 5 or older as a consequence of repeated heart infections. Usually the AV (atrioventricular) valves (see Glossary, page 114) no longer close tightly. Hardening of the tissue and scar tissue cause leaks severe enough for the blood to flow back from the ventricle into the auricle.

Effects: If the AV valve of the left side leaks, the dog develops left heart insufficiency with lung congestion and, eventually, pulmonary edema (see page 56). In right heart insufficiency, pressure builds up in the veins of the abdomen, which leads to enlargement of the liver and spleen and eventually to ascite. Chronic valvular heart disease also leads to enlargement of the heart.

● **Treatment**

➡ The veterinarian determines the nature of heart disease by listening to the heart, feeling the pulse, taking X-rays and usually an electrocardiogram. Valvular heart disease in dogs is incurable because artificial valves and their open-heart surgical implantation are too expensive. But the condition can be kept under control for years with appropriate heart medications. If fluid builds up in the lungs and the abdominal cavity, diuretics must be given.

Follow-up care: Generally, lifelong drug therapy is necessary. The drugs can easily be given in liquid form or in the form of small pills that are hidden in the food or in a treat A special low-sodium heart diet will also be prescribed.

Prevention: If there is an infection of the lungs accompanied by fever, don't rely on the self-healing powers of the body too long but take the dog to the veterinarian in good time. As a general rule, excitement, exertion, obesity, and hot, humid weather should be avoided.

■ **Homeopathy**

For dosage, see page 39.

Crataegus.

• If there is a tendency to edema and weakness of the heart muscle with inflammation of the endocardium: *Kalium carbonicum* or *Convallaria majalis.* Can also be given as supportive

treatment when the veterinarian has prescribed digitalis.

Susceptible breeds: Chronic valvular heart disease is common in old dogs of all breeds, but small- to medium-sized dogs, such as dachshunds, schnauzers, Pomeranians, poodles, and various terriers seem to be especially prone to it.

Congenital Heart Disease

There are a number of congenital heart diseases that are quite rare (they account for about 5% of all incidents of heart disease) but affect primarily certain breeds (see on right).

● **Treatment**

• Stenosis of the aorta and the pulmonary artery is generally treated with a heart stimulant (such as digitalis).

• Persistent ductus arteriosus and right arch of the aorta have to be corrected surgically. This is, however, an expensive procedure performed by veterinary surgeons with advanced training.

• Defects in the interventricular septum require open-heart surgery, during which the animal has to be connected to a heart-lung machine. The procedure is therefore used only experimentally or clinically in rare circumstances.

• Heart tumors can't as a rule be surgically removed.

Congenital Heart Diseases

• Stenosis of the aorta: Narrowing of the aorta that leads to enlargement of the left ventricle. Found primarily in boxers.

• Pulmonary stenosis: Narrowing of the pulmonary artery that leads to enlargement of the right side of the heart. Occurs in boxers, English bulldogs, beagles, fox terriers, and Chihuahuas.

• Persistent ductus arteriosus: A short connection between the aorta and the pulmonary artery just behind the heart, which causes oxygen-saturated and oxygen-depleted blood to mix. It is a remnant of embryonic and fetal circulation that normally closes soon after birth.

• Persistent right arch of the aorta: A malformation that makes the vessel press against the esophagus. Often coexists with ductus arteriosus. Found primarily in poodles, collies, German shepherds, and Labrador retrievers.

• Defects of the septum: A gap in the wall separating the left and right ventricles, allowing oxygen-saturated and oxygen-depleted blood to mix. Found in some strains of certain breeds, such as the Neapolitan mastiff.

• Heart base tumors: Found primarily in short-nosed breeds, such as boxers and Boston terriers of 5 to 6 years or older.

Inflammation of the Endocardium, Heart Muscle, and Pericardium

Symptoms: As for chronic valvular heart disease (see page 58), together with high fever.

Cause: Usually brought on by an infection of the heart valve muscle or the pericardium resulting from bacterial inflammation.

Effects:

• Inflammation of the endocardium leaves scar tissue, especially in the area of the valves, which leads to chronic heart disease.

• Inflammation of the heart muscle results—if it doesn't take an acute, fatal form—in permanent heart muscle damage with abnormalities in the heart rhythm.

• Pericarditis is often the result of chronic infections accompanied by pleurisy. The pericardium fills with fluid, thickens, and thus constrains heart action.

● **Treatment**

➡ The veterinarian tries to arrive at a precise diagnosis of the condition by taking X-rays, performing an ECG (electrocardiogram, see Glossary, page 116), perhaps taking a sample of the fluid in the pericardium, and possibly doing an ultrasound examination. It is essential to treat the underlying disease that is causing the heart condition.

Follow-up care: Defects of the cardiac valves, weakened heart muscle, and hardening of the pericardium all cause permanent organic damage that has to be treated for the rest of the dog's life with heart stimulants and, if indicated, diuretics.

Prevention: See Chronic Valvular Heart Disease, page 58.

■ **Homeopathy**

See Chronic Valvular Heart Disease, page 58.

Thrombosis, Thromboembolism, Arteriosclerosis

Diseases of the blood and lymph vessels are rare in dogs. But when they do occur they are very hard to diagnose because dogs can't communicate to us what bothers them. Observation of the symptoms is therefore especially important.

Symptoms: Sensitivity to pain in the affected area, pallor and coldness because of insufficient circulation, loss of sensation, paralysis in one or more limbs, kidney failure.

These are also symptoms of strangulation caused by too tight a bandage or by cutting off circulation to the legs.

Dizziness, staggering, absent gaze, and abnormal behavior like standing motionless or not finding the food suggest insufficient blood flow to the brain.

Causes:

• Thrombosis: Congestion of the arteries caused by blood clots, fat or connective tissue (fat embolism), inflamed cells, or foreign bodies, such as parasite larvae.

• Arteriosclerosis: This condition is found mostly in older dogs and is caused by high cholesterol and impaired fat metabolism as well as by thyroid deficiency (see page 85). The result is abnormal hardening, diminished elasticity, thickening, and constriction of blood flow.

Effects: The part of the body the congested arteries are supposed to supply with blood can no longer carry out its functions and may necrose. The signs of such malfunctionings vary, but usually are severe.

• A thrombosis or embolism of the coronary arteries brings about a heart attack, which manifests itself in a stabbing pain in the chest, shortness of breath, racing pulse, loss of consciousness, and instant death. If the thrombus is in the descending aorta, the back legs are paralyzed and the condition is often misdiagnosed as a herniated disc (see page 94). Sometimes the thromboembolism causes obstruction of blood flow to one or both kidneys.

● **Treatment**

➡ Professional help is required. The first goal is to thin the blood by means of intravenous

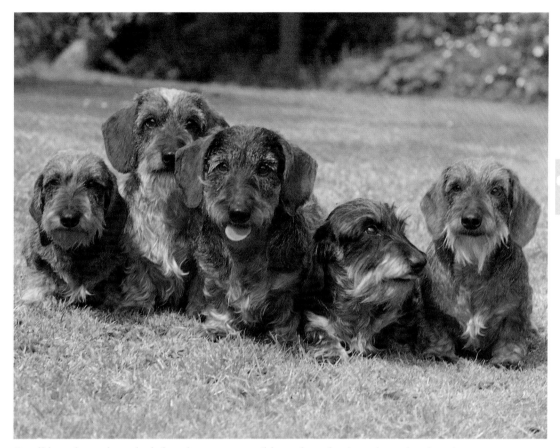

Small breeds, such as dachshunds, are susceptible to thrombosis and arteriosclerosis. Plenty of exercise and a healthy diet keep these dogs fit.

fluid therapy. Anti-coagulants can be introduced with strict monitoring.

If the blood flow to the limbs is impaired, you can help your dog by massaging it, giving it alternating hot and cold baths, and reviving circulation by rubbing stimulants, such as alcohol, into the skin. A surgical operation called an endartero-tomy can be performed to remove the clots, or a clot-dissolving drug can be infused intravenously.

Follow-up care: Drugs to stimulate blood flow to the brain, a low-fat diet (see pages 24 and 25), and perhaps heart stimulants.

Prevention: A balanced diet with reduced fat. Prevent obesi-ty, and make sure you take the dog for long walks so it gets plenty of exercise.

■ **Homeopathy**
For dosage, see page 39.
Conium maculatum.

Susceptible breeds: Mostly males of toy breeds, schnauzers, Doberman pinschers, and dachshunds.

Anemia

Anemia is a condition in which the blood is deficient in red corpuscles and/or hemoglobin, the pigment that makes the blood red and is responsible for gas exchange in the lungs.

Symptoms: Pale to white mucous membranes (observe the conjunctiva in the eyes or the inside of the lips), increased pulse rate, lack of energy, cold limbs, apathy, staggering, collapse. Depending on the underlying disease, anemia can cause bloody diarrhea, bleeding from the lining of the mouth, etc. It may be manifested by yellowish discoloration of the mucous membranes, fever, and dark urine, if the red blood cells are being destroyed in abnormally large numbers within the vascular system.

Causes: Blood loss due to injury or clotting disorders; decrease of red blood cells because of infections, parasites, poisoning, or autoimmune disorders (see pages 84 and 95); reduced production of red blood cells because of iron deficiency, severe liver or kidney disease, or damage to the bone marrow (caused by tumors, hormones, or medications).

Effects: Oxygen supply may be reduced, and the dog may be in danger of suffocating.

● **Treatment**
If there is acute bleeding caused by an injury, put a pressure bandage or tourniquet on the affected limb (see page 26) as a first-aid measure to prevent massive blood loss.

➡ Then rush the animal to the veterinarian. The most important emergency measure if there is massive blood loss is to infuse fluid into the veins. Perhaps a blood transfusion will be necessary. Dogs whose blood has been tested for compatibility can serve as donors. A precise diagnosis of chronic anemia requires special blood tests. Further treatment depends on the disease that is causing anemia.

Follow-up care and prevention: A well-balanced diet with plenty of iron (green vegetables, organ meat, and red meat are sources of iron), perhaps with an iron supplement in the form of pills. Dogs with hereditary anemia should not be bred.

Susceptible breeds: In dwarf and Doberman pinschers, Scotch terriers, golden retrievers, and German shepherds, hemophilia, a relatively rare blood disease, is found that affects only males—as in humans—but is passed on to the offspring by the female.

Blood Is a Very Special Liquid

Without blood the different parts of the body could not be supplied with all the substances they need to function. Blood consists of plasma, a fluid, and of solid bodies, the red and white blood corpuscles, and platelets responsible for blood coagulation. In the plasma there are proteins (albumins and globulins). The albumins serve primarily to nourish tissue and supply it with proteins, while the globulins play an important immune role in warding off infections. The red blood cells (erythrocytes) are responsible for the transport of oxygen and carbon dioxide, and the white blood cells (leukocytes) fight pathogens. This intricate system can be upset by diseases, with obviously serious consequences for the organism.

Leukemia

Behind this term hide a number of diseases that are sometimes referred to collectively as "cancer of the blood" and lead—as in humans—to serious general symptoms with tumorous growths all over the body, the internal organs, and the skeletal system.

Symptoms: Depending on the nature of the growth, the organs it primarily affects, and the extent to which it has spread, the symptoms can vary a great deal. In the most common kinds of "blood cancer" they are:

• Lymphatic leukemia: Swelling of the lymph nodes to enormous size, especially on the throat. This cancer spreads to the internal organs (see Metastasis, Glossary, page 118), attacking the lungs, intestines, liver, or spleen and causing apathy, lack of appetite, emaciation, anemia, jaundice, bleeding of the mucous membranes (lips), vomiting, diarrhea, and complete debility.

Causes: "Blood cancer" is caused by abnormalities and growths in the blood-producing tissue of the lymph nodes (lymphatic leukemia) and the bone marrow (myeloid leukemia), as well as in other tissues since the blood and lymph system extends throughout the body and internal organs (lymphoma).

Effects: Blood cancer is almost always malignant and generally incurable, although many dogs will live relatively normal lives if treated with appropriate chemotherapy by trained veterinary oncologists.

● **Treatment**
➡ Professional help is required.
• Lymphatic leukemia seems to respond in the very early stages to cortisone and anticancer chemotherapeutic drugs (see Glossary, page 115). But the disease is only rarely completely cured.

• All other forms of blood cancer are much rarer in dogs than in humans and seem at this time to be incurable, especially if they are not caught at an early stage.

Follow-up care: If lymphatic leukemia has responded to treatment, regular check-ups every 1 to 3 months are imperative.

Tumors of the Spleen

Symptoms: Apathy, anemia (pale mucous membranes), increase in the size of the belly, light fever. The belly is usually somewhat taut and sensitive to touch.

Causes: Tumors of the spleen are most commonly the consequence of growths on the blood vessels. A sudden increase in the size of the belly suggests bleeding from a tumor.

Effects: Tumors of the spleen are usually malignant and in a high percentage of the cases spread to the liver, lungs, heart, or kidneys. If there is internal bleeding, the dog can bleed to death.

● **Treatment**
➡ Professional help is required.
Through blood tests, X-rays of the abdomen and lungs, and a biopsy, diagnosis is possible. If

The Spleen — An Important Organ

Next to the bone marrow, the spleen is the most important blood generating organ. The spleen also holds 10% of the blood and fulfills many functions in the filtering, cleaning, and regeneration of blood. Being so involved with blood, it is especially vulnerable to cancer.

the cancer has not yet spread to the lungs, the spleen can be removed, since its functions will be taken over by the bone marrow, liver, and lymph system.

If the spleen is removed because of a tear in it, because of non-malignant growths, or because of a torsion (twisting) (usually in large dogs), the chances of recovery are good. Intravenous injection of fluids and perhaps blood transfusions are necessary during the operation.

Follow-up care: Antibiotics for 1 week to ward off peritonitis.

Prevention: If malignant tumors are surgically removed, regular check-ups every 1 to 3 months are recommended.

Disorders of the Urinary Tract and the Genital Organs

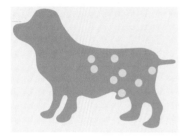

*W*hen you take your dog for a walk and it wants to stop and lift its leg at every tree you pass, this may seem an annoying habit to you, but for the dog it is the equivalent of our writing letters. The urine the dog is distributing is produced by the kidneys, the vital organs that filter many toxic substances from the blood. From the kidneys the urine travels through the ureter and collects in the bladder, and from there it passes through the urethra and is voided. The genital organs are connected to the urinary tract.

Acute Urinary Tract and Bladder Infection

Symptoms: Urine is bloody and cloudy, sometimes mixed with mucus; occasionally there are gravelly stones and clotted blood in it; urgency to void; either frequent urinating that may be accompanied by expressions of pain or attempts to void that yield nothing or only a few drops.

Causes: Usually the infection is caused by bacteria and travels up the urinary tract. Because the urethra is shorter in females, they are prone to bladder infections. But older males, which often have enlarged and chronically inflamed prostate, tend to suffer from chronic bladder and kidney problems, too (see page 66).

● Treatment

Make sure the dog takes in enough liquids (this helps dilute the urine and flush out the system); mix concentrates of bladder and kidney tea (available from health food stores) into the drinking water or, more effectively, mix the powder into the food.
➡ If there is no rapid improvement, take the dog to the veterinarian. Laboratory analysis of the urine is used for diagnosis. Antibiotics and sulfa drugs (see Glossary, pages 114 and 119) are effective against blad-

der infections (cystitis), which are usually caused by bacteria.

Follow-up care: Give antibiotics for 1 week and add bladder and kidney tea as well as salt to the food to increase thirst and thus increase water consumption.

■ Homeopathy

For dosage, see page 39.
Solidago.
• If the urine is yellow, opaque, and with flakes of matter: *Berberis.*
• If frequent urination yields only a few drops at a time: *Cantharis.*

Stones in the Urinary Tract

Symptoms: Bloody urine, sometimes with gravelly grit; constant urge to void; dribbling of urine, or refusal to urinate.

Causes: Bladder infections can give rise to small stones that may later grow to the size of plums and irritate the bladder wall, leading to constant bleeding in the bladder. Especially in male dogs, small stones cause urinating problems because they can lodge in the urethra, thus obstructing the urine flow.

● Treatment

➡ Take the dog to the veterinarian, who can diagnose the problem by X-raying the bladder, which first has to have air introduced into it. Small bladder stones can be flushed out by rinsing the bladder or with a loop catheter. If no urine at all is passed, immediate surgery is imperative because the bladder might otherwise burst. Larger bladder or kidney stones also have to be operated on.

Follow-up care: Antibiotics are given until the urine is normal again, which can take 3 to 4 weeks in old males. In addition, feed a special diet designed to prevent bladder stones (available from your veterinarian). Add some salt to the food (1–5 grams per day) to make the dog increase its intake of liquids.

Prevention: There are special drugs and diets to prevent renewed formation of all kinds of urinary stones. The veterinarian will prescribe an appropriate one.

Susceptible breeds: Dalmatians, dachshunds, poodles, German shepherds, boxers, pugs, and Irish and Cairn terriers tend to develop various kinds of urinary stones.

Urinating Disorders

Symptoms: Uncontrolled passing of urine (incontinence), dribbling, or refusal to urinate.

Causes: Overly full bladder, nervous disorder after herniated discs, scarring and other tissue abnormalities, behavioral problems, weakness of the sphincter muscles in stressful situations. Incontinence is most often seen in older dogs, especially in spayed females.

● Treatment

➡ Take the dog to the veterinarian. If the problem is hormonal, females are treated with low doses of estrogen and males are given androgen. However, newer drugs, such as phenylpropanolamine have fewer side effects and may be used instead. In addition ephedrine may be given to lower the response threshold of the muscle closing the bladder.

■ Homeopathy

For dosage, see page 39.

Dulcamara, Petroselinum, Uva ursi, Solidago, and *Natrium choratum* are given in combination.

Susceptible breeds: Incontinence due primarily to hormonal causes is more common in older females of all larger breeds if they were spayed at a young age. Among these breeds are Great Danes, Dobermans, boxers, German shepherds, and sheep dogs.

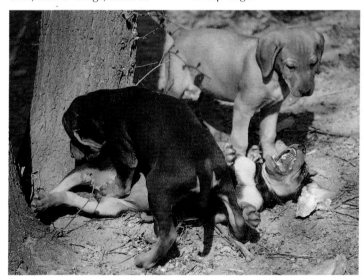

Puppies often lose control over the muscles of the urinary sphincter when they get excited. This is normal and will cease later.

Acute Kidney Failure

Symptoms: Little or no urine output; later, increased thirst. The urine that is passed is usually darker than normal or even bloody, the loin area hurts, and the belly is distended. Fever only if there is an inflammation. Vomiting, even when the stomach is empty, and a sour, urine-like smell from the mouth. Apathetic behavior, refusal to eat.

Causes: Acute kidney failure can be caused by
• shock and major blood loss caused by an accident;
• extensive vomiting and diarrhea;
• serious infections in the abdomen, such as peritonitis and pyometra;
• poisoning with heavy metals (mercury, lead, arsenic, cadmium, and thallium, which is found primarily in rat poison), or antifreeze (glycol);
• retention of urine because of stones in the bladder or urethra or because of an injured urethra or a tear in the bladder.

Effects: Acute kidney failure can be fatal.

● **Treatment**
➡ Rush the animal to the veterinarian. Acute kidney failure is an emergency and has to be treated aggressively. The dog is hooked up to an intravenous line and given diuretics to start the kidneys working again.

Then the cause of kidney failure has to be determined and treated.

Follow-up care: Treatment of the underlying disease, such as bacterial pyelonephritis, with antibiotics over a period of several weeks. Also a strict kidney diet (see page 24).

■ **Homeopathy**
For dosage, see page 39.
Apis, Berberis, Solidago, Veratrum, Juniperus communis, Galium album, phosphorus.

Chronic Kidney Disease

Symptoms: Increased thirst and urine output, vomiting (also of blood), stool often dark and soft, weight loss, shaggy coat, urine smell from the mouth, apathy, below-normal temperature, dazed state or heightened excitability.

Causes: Accumulated damage to kidney tissue from previous inflammations and infectious diseases (such as leptospirosis, see page 99), as well as several other diseases lead to chronic kidney disease (see Kidney Diseases, page 67).

Effects: Uremic poisoning; decalcification of the bones (through increased phosphorus level in the blood, which causes calcium loss) leading to osteoporosis (osteorenal syndrome).

● **Treatment**
➡ Visit the veterinarian immediately. Diagnosis is based on blood analyses that reveal urea, creatinine, and phosphorus levels. Infusion of appropriate substances, such as sodium and diuretics can stimulate the kidneys to start excreting urine again. Tablets and liquids containing aluminum hydroxyde bind phosphorus. A kidney diet (see page 24) is also important to keep the kidneys functioning. In acute cases, the body has to be detoxified by peritoneal dialysis.

Follow-up care: Kidney diet for life. Ensure adequate intake of liquids by giving the dog diluted skim milk to drink and adding salt to the food (1–5 grams per day); add concentrate of bladder and kidney tea to the drinking water or mix it in powder form into the food.

■ **Homeopathy**
See under Acute Kidney Failure, this page.

Kidney Diseases

The following diseases lead to chronic kidney damage.

• Glomerulonephritis (inflammation of the glomeruli, the small masses of tissue at the base of each nephron): Impairment of renal function resulting in the elimination of important protein substances.

• Pyelonephritis (inflammation of the kidneys and the renal pelvis): Bacterial inflammation of kidney tissue and the renal pelvis.

• Kidney amyloidosis (highly acute or chronic inflammation of the kidney tissue): Deposit of fibrous protein particles in the glomeruli. Presumably caused in part by autoimmune reactions (see pages 84 and 95).

• Cystic kidneys: Congenital or inherited malformation of kidney tissue, which prevents urine from flowing off and results in empty cyst-like "bubbles" in the kidneys.

Hydronephrosis (retention of urine in the renal pelvis): Malformations or blockage of the outflow (tumors, kidney stones) and the consequent pressure of retained urine result in a widening, thinning, and ballooning of the renal pelvis and atrophy of kidney tissue.

Kidney tumors: Destruction of renal tissue and likelihood of metastasis (see Glossary, page 118) to other organs.

Prostate Problems

Symptoms: Difficulty passing stool; frequent urge to defecate; sometimes blood and pus in the urine; also fever and acute pain in the abdomen.

Causes: Obstruction of the rectum caused by the enlarged prostate gland. This condition frequently affects older males (7 years and older) and is enhanced by male sex hormone. Often the prostate gland is not only enlarged but inflamed as well.

Effects: An enlarged prostate gland can lead to chronic kidney and bladder inflammations and to abscesses and cysts. The straining involved in passing stool sometimes causes a hernia (see Hernia, page 49).

● **Treatment**
Try first to relieve the discomfort associated with defecating by giving the dog easily digestible food (see Diets, pages 24 and 25).

➡ If the dog has a fever, see the veterinarian. The prostate gland, normally the size of a walnut, can grow as big as an apple. Estrogen treatments shrink the gland only temporarily. Neutering (see Glossary, page 118) is recommended as a permanent solution. If the inflammation is necrotizing, give pain relievers and antibiotics; if abscessed or cystic, surgery is usually required.

Follow-up care: To prevent the infection from spreading to the kidneys, antibiotics should be given for 2 to 3 weeks to combat cystitis, which usually goes along with prostate enlargement.

Prevention: The best way to avoid prostate problems is to neuter older males. This reduces the size of the prostate gland. Castrated dogs don't become lazy and inactive, as many people think, but they do like to eat more. Make sure your neutered dog doesn't get obese because excess weight does make dogs less active. If necessary, reduce the meals to half or a third of the previous amount (see Weight Loss Diet, page 25).

■ **Homeopathy**
For dosage, see page 39.
• For swelling of the prostate gland: *Magnesium carbonicum, Magnesium chloratium, Magnesium phosphoricum, Thuja, Sabal serrulatum.*
• For inflammation: *Pulsatilla, Thuja, Bryonia.*
• If there is a complication involving the spinal column in the groin and sacrum area: *Colocynthis.*

Inflammation of the Testicles (Orchitis)

Symptoms: Swelling and reddening of one or both testicles; painful response to touch; sometimes fever and refusal to eat. Stiff gait with somewhat straddled hind legs.

Causes: Injuries and contusions. Infection caused by bacteria.

Effects: Formation of putrid abscesses in the testicles.

● Treatment
You should treat acute inflammations of the scrotum with lukewarm camomile baths and application of a zinc ointment, which you can get from your veterinarian or a drugstore.
➡ If there is a purulent infection, take the dog to the veterinarian. He or she will prescribe antibiotics in tablet form, which have to be taken for 1 week or more. A soothing ointment may be prescribed.

Follow-up care: Bathe the area with a camomile solution 2 or 3 times a day, then apply a zinc ointment. Continue this until the inflammation subsides. An Elizabethan collar (see page 22) will have to be put on the dog because the sores will not heal if the dog licks them.

■ Homeopathy
For dosage, see page 39.
For eczema on the scrotum: *Croton.*

Testicular Tumors

Symptoms: Lopsidedly enlarged testes are quite normal in dogs 6 years old or older. But if one or both testicles become enlarged within a short time, this is a warning signal. Hair loss and itching all over, enlarged nipples, and general change to a more female appearance suggest a testicular tumor in the abdomen.

Causes and effects: Tumors tend to form on malformed testes. In the course of a male puppy's development the testicles normally descend out of the abdominal cavity. Sometimes, because of hereditary factors, they remain in the abdominal cavity or in the groin area (cryp-torchidism). When these dogs reach the age of 5 to 7 years, their testicles tend to grow indiscriminately and secrete mostly female hormones.

Tumors in normally positioned testicles usually lead to prostate problems.

● Treatment
➡ Take the dog to the vet. Either kind of tumor should be operated on as soon as possible since both are sometimes malignant.

Prevention: Remove cryptorchid testicles surgically by the time the dog is 2 years old, before they turn problematic.

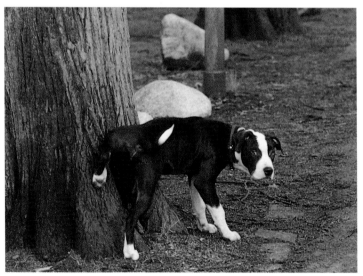

Excessive marking and frequent roaming can be a sign of hypersexuality.

Hypersexuality

Symptoms: Aggressive behavior, attempts to mount people and cushions, excessive roaming and marking of territory.

Causes: Overproduction of male hormones that may be triggered by testicular tumors (see page 68).

Effects: Inflammation of the foreskin and prostate problems (see page 67) especially in old age.

● **Treatment**

➡ The veterinarian will try to reduce the male's sexual urge by prescribing estrogen, especially while bitches in the neighborhood are in heat. To take care of the problem permanently, castration is recommended (see Glossary, page 115).

Inability to Mate and Infertility

Symptoms: Unsuccessful attempts at mating, premature exhaustion after a few attempts to copulate.

Causes: Malnutrition or obesity; circulatory problems; weak hind quarters; hormonal malfunctioning; diseases of the genital organs; also psychic causes, such as inexperience in the male or lack of ease in an unfamiliar setting.

● **Treatment**

A well-balanced diet (see pages 12–15) is always recommended. Nervous males have to be introduced to an unfamiliar environment gradually, and sometimes help is needed guiding the penis into the vagina.

➡ In cases of infertility the veterinarian will examine the semen to determine the number of spermatozoa, their normal appearance, and their mobility. Inflammations, infections, and cryptorchidism (see Testicular Tumors, page 68) can cause infertility. Antibiotics can often cure the problem if it is due to inflammation of the testicles. Hormone treatments, on the other hand, are not very promising except in young males.

Susceptible breeds: In some English strains of the pit bull terrier, the male occasionally attacks the bitch instead of mounting her. Here the aggressive drive seems to win out over the instinct to perpetuate the species. These individuals automatically eliminate themselves from the breeding stock.

Young, inexperienced males sometimes have difficulties mating. If necessary, provide some assistance.

Vaginal Infection

Symptoms: Purulent, and sometimes bloody or mucoid vaginal discharge; excessive licking of the vulva; outer folds of the vagina large and swollen, sometimes with protrusion of the vagina (vaginal prolapse); dragging the rear end along the ground (see Scooting, Glossary, page 118).

Causes: Bacterial infection of the vagina (vaginitis), occasionally occurs very early, even before the first heat cycle. The germs are transmitted during copulation. Vaginal prolapse occurs primarily in large females during heat. Vaginal tumors.

Effects: A severe case of vaginitis can lead to uterine disease (see page 72).

● Treatment

➡ The dog should be thoroughly examined by the veterinarian, who will irrigate the vagina every 2 days with a mild disinfectant using a douche. If the discharge is purulent, antibiotics are given to get rid of the germs. Vaginal prolapse, injuries, and tumors usually require surgery. Recurrent vaginal prolapse is best dealt with by spaying (see Glossary, page 119).

Follow-up care: Clean the labia majora of all traces of discharge 2 to 3 times daily with a cotton ball dipped in baby oil or witch hazel.

Susceptible breeds: Vaginal prolapse during heat is seen primarily in large breeds, such as Great Danes, Saint Bernards, and Bernese mountain dogs.

Mastitis

Symptoms: A watery, blood-tinged secretion can be expressed from the nipple if pressure is put on the breasts. Affected glands are swollen, painful, and warm to the touch. Fever.

Causes: Bacterial infection of a mammary gland that usually has been previously damaged by coagulated milk or injuries inflicted by nursing puppies.

Effects: Formation of abscesses on the mammary organ.

● Treatment

In a light case of mastitis you can massage the breast with rubbing alcohol (50%) or a

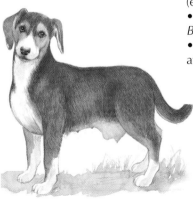

camphorated ointment to stimulate circulation and cool the area.

➡ If there is a bloody and purulent secretion, the dog must be taken to the vet. It is probably suffering from bacterial mastitis and must be given antibiotics. Swollen and hard abscesses may have to be lanced under anesthesia.

Follow-up care: Antibiotics must always be given for an entire week. After the abscess has been lanced, the wound should be drained (see Glossary, page 116) for 3 to 4 days and kept covered with a bandage. The puppies must be bottle fed and not permitted to nurse on the affected bitch.

Prevention: Check the teats of a nursing dog regularly because a putrescent infection can spread to the puppies.

■ Homeopathy

For dosage, see page 39.

Apis, belladonna, Aconitum (especially in the early stages).
● If the dog is very thirsty: *Bryonia.*
● If the dog's general health is affected: *Echinacea angustifolia.*

Tumors on the mammary glands most commonly turn up on the posterior glands.

Breast Tumors

Symptoms: Lumps in the breast, sometimes flat and occasionally ulcerating at the surface.

Causes: About half of all the tumors in female dogs originate in the mammary glands. Old intact (non-spayed) females (average age 9 years) tend to develop breast tumors. Frequent pregnancies or constant false pregnancy (see page 72) increases the tumor risk. Regular hormone shots to prevent estrus also increase the risk of mammary, ovarian, and uterine cancer.

● **Treatment**
➡ The veterinarian determines whether or not a biopsied tumor is malignant by analyzing a tissue sample. Small lumps (less than ¼ inch or 5 mm in diameter) are at first monitored, larger ones are surgically removed. If there is reason to think that the lumps are malignant, the tissue around them and sometimes all the breasts on one side have to be removed. Before such radical surgery is undertaken, a chest X-ray should be taken to make sure the cancer hasn't already spread to the lungs, in which case it is too late for operating.

Follow-up care: Sometimes a body bandage is necessary so that the incision can heal.

Prevention of Breast Tumors

If you have an older female, feel each breast all over whenever you pet her. This way you will discover in good time lumps that might be forming. A check-up by the veterinarian twice a year is also recommended.

Early spaying—the best time is between the first and the second heat—also reduces the chance of breast tumors (by 75%).

Failure to Develop Estrus (Anestrus)

Symptoms: The female skips a heat cycle but shows no signs of illness.

Causes: Hormonal malfunctioning usually originating in the ovaries or pituitary gland. Sometimes also occurs after hormones are given to prevent heat.

● **Treatment**
If you don't care about having puppies there is no need to treat anestrus.
➡ If you do want offspring from your dog, the veterinarian will prescribe hormone treatments to stimulate the production of sexual hormones. The best times for this are spring and fall (the normal heat seasons). Treatments are successful in a variable percentage of cases.

■ **Homeopathy**
For dosage, see page 39.
Aristolochia, Pulsatilla, Apis, Sepia. The same remedies can be given to females with an excessive sexual drive (nymphomania).

Prolonged Estrus

Symptoms: Vaginal discharge, swollen vulva, shedding, dull and ragged coat, itching.

Causes: Hormonal disorders originating in the ovaries or the pituitary gland. Excessive secretion in the uterus caused by continuous hormone production from ovarian cysts or tumors or by repeated hormone treatments to prevent pregnancy.

Effects: Endometritis or pyometra (see page 72).

● **Treatment**
➡ Only a veterinarian can determine whether or not prolonged estrus has already turned into endometritis. Hormonal treatments prescribed to stop vaginal bleeding can result in endometritis. The best solution is spaying.

3

71

Endometritis and Pyometra

Symptoms: Purulent, foul smelling vaginal discharge (but not always); increased thirst; about 6 to 10 weeks after estrus sometimes lethargy, fever, poor appetite, vomiting, weakness in the hind quarters; gradual increase in girth.

Causes: Hormonal disorders or hormones given to prevent estrus and pregnancy can cause uterine inflammation (endometritis) and infection (pyometra).

Effects: Liver and kidney disease, also peritonitis.

● **Treatment**

➡ Take the dog to the veterinarian immediately. If the disease is still at an early stage or if there is heavy vaginal discharge, noninvasive treatment with antibiotics and hormones (prostaglandins) for at least 1 week can be tried. However, in most cases a hysterectomy is unavoidable. If an enlarged uterus has already caused severe kidney damage and uremia, the operation becomes much more dangerous. The dog has to receive intravenous fluid therapy to improve kidney function before the operation.

Follow-up care: Antibiotics for at least 1 week or, if there is kidney disease, for 2 to 3 weeks or more.

Prevention: Early spaying is the best prevention. Spaying not only prevents uterine inflammation and infection but also lessens the chance of mammary tumors.

■ **Homeopathy**

For dosage, see page 39.

Pulsatilla, Lachesis, Echinacea angustifolia, Apis, phosphorus, *Sepia, Aconitum.*
• During convalescence after a hysterectomy: *Sabina* (to help eliminate the pus remaining in the stump of the uterus).

False Pregnancy

Symptoms: Enlargement of the breasts about 6 to 8 weeks after estrus. If pressure is applied, the nipples secrete milk. Nest building; defending of toys; aggressive behavior; hiding; lack of or, sometimes, increased appetite.

Causes: Even females that didn't conceive during estrus undergo a kind of hormonal pregnancy, which can lead to milk production after about 2 months, the time the puppies would be due. This made good sense when dogs were still living wild and females lactating because of false pregnancy could nurse puppies from large litters. Under conditions of domestication, however, these dogs have no chance to act as surrogate mothers, and their health suffers.

Effects: If the milk is not extracted, the mammary glands become inflamed.

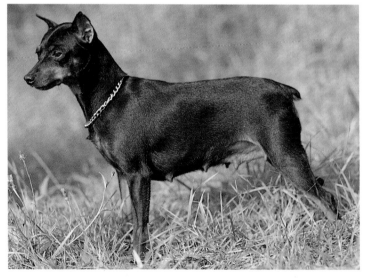

A bitch undergoing false pregnancy has enlarged nipples that may even produce milk.

● **Treatment**
Massage the breasts with diluted alcohol or salves that stimulate circulation. This helps the swelling go down faster and discourages inflammation. Try to distract the disoriented bitch by taking her on walks. Remove blankets and other nest building material as well as toys, which are often adopted as surrogate puppies.
➡ If the breasts become inflamed, take the dog to the veterinarian, who will extract the milk but only from the congested glands. For serious inflammation anti-inflammatory drugs (see Glossary, page 114) and, sometimes, antibiotics have to be given. A series of injections (twice daily for 4 to 6 days) can stop the milk production, but dogs often react with vomiting. False pregnancy normally lasts only 2 to 3 weeks.
Follow-up care: Prevent inflammation of the mammary glands by massaging them and continue taking the dog for walks to get her mind off nest building.
Prevention: If you don't want your dog to have any more

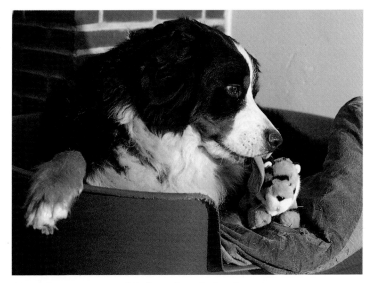

In a false pregnancy, bitches often "adopt" toys as surrogate puppies. You should remove these toys as soon as you can.

puppies, have her spayed (see Glossary, page 119). A bitch that can't get pregnant also can't develop false pregnancy. In addition, spaying lessens the risk of lumps and tumors in the breasts.

■ **Homeopathy**
For dosage, see page 39.
• The following remedies given in combination act as a prophy-lactic against false pregnancy. Start giving them 3 weeks after estrus ends. *Apis, Ammonium bromatum,* palladium, *Platinum metallicum, Mellilotus, Moschus, Sepia, Ingnatia, Aquilegia vulgaris, Cypripedium pubescens, Majorana.*
• If false pregnancy has already developed: *Asafoetida, Ignatia, Thuja, Pulsatilla, Lachesis, Moschus.*

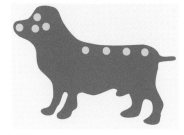

Disorders of the Sensory Organs

*D*ogs are famous for their noses. They can not only smell where people are buried in an avalanche but also sniff out the most ingeniously hidden caches of illegal drugs. We don't appreciate their love for putrid smells quite as much. Nothing seems to be as delicious to a dog as feces or a smelly old bone. Not to mention the intriguing perfumes emitted by the anal glands during mutual sniffing.

Conjunctivitis

Symptoms: Inflammation of the conjunctiva; increased tearing; sensitivity to light; thickened and bulging third eyelid (nictating membrane, see drawing, page 75); swelling of eyelids because of rubbing the eyes with the paws. These symptoms are common in almost all disorders of the eyes.

Causes: Wind, dust, congestion of the lachrymal canals, allergies, infections, caustic liquids, foreign bodies in the eyes (dirt particles, sand).

Effects: Chronic conjunctivitis, often combined with small blisters on the nictating membrane.

● Treatment

If the conjunctiva are irritated and there is a clear secretion, clean the eyelids 2 to 3 times a day with lukewarm water or camomile solution. Put anti-irritant eye drops (available from the veterinarian or a drugstore) into the eye 3 or 4 times.
➡ A mucoid and purulent discharge indicates a bacterial infection that should be treated by the veterinarian. Eye ointments containing antibiotics and cortisone are most effective. Foreign bodies are usually located beneath the lower lid or behind the nictating membrane and usually can be removed only under anesthesia. Anesthesia is usually also necessary for treating blisters of the nictating membrane.

Follow-up care: Apply eye drops 4 to 6 times and ointment 2 to 3 times daily (see Care of a Sick Dog, page 23). Clean sticky or encrusted eyelids regularly.

Prevention: Don't expose the dog to drafts and keep it from getting its head dirty.

Susceptible breeds: All dogs with long, bushy hair on the head that can reach and irritate the eyes. For example, Yorkshire terriers, Shih Tzus, poodles, Maltese, and Pekingese. German shepherds and collies tend to develop growths on the conjunctiva and third eyelid that require permanent treatment with cortisone and eye ointments containing antibiotics.

■ Homeopathy for Eye Disorders

For dosage, see page 39.
• For slightly protruding third eyelid: *Graphites* and *Causticum.*
• For swollen eyelids: *Apis.*
• For purulent eyelids and severe tear flow: *Rhus toxicodendron.*
• For follicular conjunctivitis (irritated, grainy looking eye membranes): *Staphisagria.*
• For superficial inflammation of the cornea: *Kalium bichromaticum.*

Disorders of the Eyelids

Symptoms: See Conjunctivitis, page 74.

Causes and effects:
• Eye slit too narrow with lid rolled inward (entropion): eyelashes and hair irritate the eyes (dystichiasis).
• Eye slit too wide with lower lid rolled outward (ectropion): Infections in the eyes.
• Small, purulent pimples caused by inflammation of sebacious glands along margin of eyelids.
• Larger and harder pustules (sties) growing from glands on inside of lids.

Both of the above gland problems give rise to suppurating conjunctivitis (see page 74).

● **Treatment**
➡ Take the dog to the veterinarian. Don't try to squeeze the pus from pimples or sties yourself. You will only cause the dog needless pain and may cause the infection to spread. Usually surgery is necessary.

Follow-up care and prevention: See Conjunctivitis, page 74.

■ **Homeopathy**
See page 74.

Susceptible breeds: Entropion occurs primarily in chows, hounds, and Shar Peis; ectropion, in Saint Bernards, bassets, spaniels, Bernese mountain dogs, mastiffs, Great Danes, and boxers.

Adenoma of the Third Eyelid

Symptoms: Pink, roundish lump at the nasal corner of the eye; severe tearing.

Causes: Growth on the lymphoid gland beneath the third eyelid that causes the lid to bulge out or that pops out beyond the lid (see drawing).

● **Treatment**
➡ This condition must be surgically treated by the veterinarian.
Follow-up care: Eye drops 4 to 6 times and eye ointment 2 to 3 times daily. Continued regular cleaning of the lids is important.

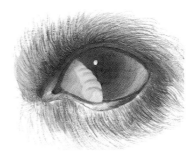

Prolapsed third eyelid with glandular growth.

Inflammation of the Cornea

Symptoms: Cloudy or milky opaqueness of the cornea. Inflammation of the cornea (keratitis) is usually accompanied by conjunctivitis (see page 74).

Causes: Mechanical irritation caused by hairs, lashes, or foreign bodies and bacterial infections produce clouding of the cornea, in which small ulcers can develop.

Effects: If the ulcers penetrate the cornea, the eye may be lost.

● **Treatment**
Visit the veterinarian immediately because this condition is potentially sight-threatening. Antibiotic eye ointments with added cortisone can relieve corneal inflammation, but since cortisone can cause ulceration, careful dosage is crucial.

Larger ulcers are scraped off the cornea under anesthesia and treated with a mild iodine tincture. Often a piece of conjunctiva or nictating membrane is sewn over the ulcer to prevent the eye from collapsing and being lost.

Follow-up care: Antibiotic eye drops (4–6 times daily) and eye ointments (2–3 times daily), sometimes for several weeks.

■ **Homeopathy**
See page 74.

Susceptible breeds: Chronic inflammation of the cornea (congenital) is found primarily in German shepherds but also occurs in collies, Saint Bernards, and dachshunds. All short-nosed breeds, such as boxers, pugs, Boston terriers, French bulldogs, and especially Pekingese tend to develop keratitis and corneal ulceration. In Pekingese, the hairs growing from the nose folds tend to prick the eyes (often the nose fold has to be surgically removed).

Cataracts

Symptoms: Milky to bluish opacity of the lens, dilated pupil, but frequently no obvious, acute symptoms, such as tearing.

Causes: Cataracts are in most cases hereditary, but they can also be brought on by other disorders of the eye, such as retinal atrophy, prolapsed lens, and serious infections or injuries of the eye. Diabetes always causes cataracts in old age.

Effects: Gradual blindness as the cataract grows. Development of glaucoma.

● **Treatment**
➡ Consult the veterinarian. Some animal clinics perform cataract surgery in which the lens is removed or replaced with an implant. But this operation is necessary only if both eyes are affected because a cataract in one eye is no prob-

lem for a dog as long as it is not likely to lead to glaucoma.

Follow-up care: The dog has to be kept stationary and have the head bandage changed daily. An Elizabethan collar is necessary so that the eye can heal undisturbed.

Prevention: Many products are available, but none of them are effective because in most cases cataracts are hereditary or are due to old age.

Susceptible breeds: Cataracts are the most widespread hereditary disorder in dogs. Most breeds are susceptible, but cataracts are most prevalent in poodles, spaniels, golden and Labrador retrievers, schnauzers, bull terriers, and collies.

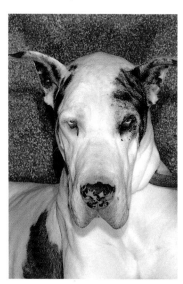

Great Dane suffering from conjunctivitis.

Retinal Atrophy

Symptoms: The first sign is night blindness, followed by diminishing eyesight in daytime and dilated pupils.

Causes: Hereditary disorder; progressve retinal atrophy (PRA).

Effects: Eventual loss of sight.

● **Treatment**
➡ Only a veterinarian can properly diagnose the condition.

The retina is a layer of light-sensitive cells in the back of the eye and can be examined only with a special illuminated instrument. The disorder is incurable, and only the complications, such as conjunctivitis (page 74), can be treated.

Follow-up care: Apply 2 to 3 times daily an ointment that suppresses inflammation.

Prevention: Dogs with hereditary progressive retinal atrophy should be excluded from breeding. This is now being done in the case of some breeds, but PRA doesn't manifest itself until the age of 3 to 5 years, when a dog may already have produced or sired several litters.

Susceptible breeds: Especially common in toy poodles, some kinds of spaniels, Bernese mountain dogs, Irish setters, toy and long-haired dachshunds, and Tibetan terriers.

Glaucoma

Symptoms: Bulging, enlarged eye ball with dilated pupil, through which the retina appears greenish. Excessive tearing and considerable inflammation of the entire eye.

Causes: Cataracts and retinal atrophy both cause the pupils to dilate so more light can enter the eye. The dilation impedes the flow of fluid from the eye chamber and thus causes pressure inside the eye to build up. Other causes of glaucoma are injuries, inflammation, and tumors.

● **Treatment**
➡ The veterinarian can prescribe drugs for temporary relief of the pressure and to reduce the intraocular fluid in the eye, but only surgical intervention offers permanent relief. If the glaucoma is incurable, the eyeball may have to be removed.

Infections of the Outer Ear

Symptoms: Head shaking and tilting of the head, scratching the ears, sometimes a foul smelling discharge, painful reaction to touch.

Causes: Water in the ear, excessive ear wax production, ear mites, fungi, warts, tumors, injuries, foreign bodies.

● **Treatment**
➡ A precise diagnosis by the

■ **Homeopathy for Ear Infections**
For dosage, see page 39.
• Severe itching: *Mercurius solubilis.*
• Dry, inflamed ear: Petroleum, sulfur.
• Excessive ear wax: *Graphites silicea.*
• Yellowish brown discharge: *Psorinum,* sulfur.
• Yellowish, thick, and foul smelling discharge mixed with blood and pus: *Hepar sulfuris.*
• Runny, caustic discharge: *belladonna.*
• If warts in addition to any of the above: *Causticum.*
• Light cases of swollen ear flap: Massage the ear with Traumeel ointment.

veterinarian is necessary. There are medications against ear mites and ticks (brownish black discharge), ear drops containing antibiotics to fight bacteria, and antimycotic drugs (see Glossary, page 114). Irrigations of the ear (performed under anesthesia) are the most effective treatment. Foreign bodies are removed with special forceps. The dog is usually anesthesized for this as well as for surgical removal of warts and tumors. If a dog has chronic ear problems, often the only solution is an operation in which the deeper part of the ear canal is opened up. Afterwards infections heal quickly.

Follow-up care: Apply ear drops daily after cleaning the ears (see Ear Care, page 18). Take the dog to the veterinarian for weekly check-ups until the ear is completely healed.

Prevention: Regular, monthly cleaning of the ears.

Susceptible breeds: Drop-eared breeds, like spaniels, setters, bloodhounds, and bassets, tend to have narrow ear canals and to form a lot of ear wax. Thick hair in the ear canal, often found in poodles, terriers, and in wooly mongrels, also encourages ear infections.

Swollen Ear Flap

Symptoms: Sudden swelling of the ear flap with fluid inside.

Causes: Accumulation of blood between the skin and the cartilage of the ear. Dogs with ear infections tend to scratch and shake their heads violently, which results in broken blood vessels and bleeding.

Effects: Scarring and shriveling of the ear.

● **Treatment**
➡ Puncturing and drawing off the fluid with a syringe to reduce swelling, but this rarely brings permanent relief. Generally an operation is necessary in which the ear flap is sewn between two gauze-padded plastic shields.

Follow-up care: Head bandage for 1 week; remove sutures at end of second week. Treat cause.

4

Disorders of the Skin and the Endocrine Glands

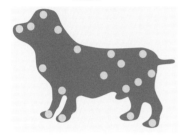

*T*he coat is what keeps a dog warm and what, whether the hair is short and smooth or long and curly, makes it look beautiful. Beneath the fur is the skin, the body's largest organ in terms of area. A dog's skin is tough; it prevents dehydration, protects against injury, and acts as a barrier against pathogens. It conveys pain as well as the physical pleasure of being petted. It is loose and elastic. The only thing a dog's skin can't do is sweat. Dogs regulate body heat primarily by panting.

Hair Loss

Symptoms: Hairless spots of varying size up to complete nakedness.

Causes and Effects:
• Scratching or biting to relieve severe itching caused by fleas or an allergy usually results not only in hair loss but also in sores.
• Mite infestation.
• Not enough zinc or essential fatty acids in the food.
• Serious illnesses and stressful conditions, such as worm infestations, general infection accompanied by fever, the strain of giving birth and nursing puppies.
• Hormonal imbalances often lead to symmetrical hair loss in the kidney region, on the thighs, or on the entire body.
• Ringworm (caused by fungi) shows up as circular bare spots on which the skin turns dark.
• Poisoning with thallium (ingredient of rat poison) or cytostatic (cancer chemotherapeutic) drugs (see Glossary, page 115) can cause complete hair loss.
• Hereditary hairlessness as a breeding goal: hairless breeds, such as the Mexican Hairless and Chinese Crested.

● **Treatment**
➡ Through laboratory analysis of skin scrapings, checking of hormone levels in the blood, or skin biopsies, the veterinarian can establish the cause of the problem. Then the disease, parasite infestation, allergy, infection, hormonal malfunctioning, or other causative factor has to be treated (see following pages).
    Follow-up care, prevention: A balanced diet (see pages 12 and 15) is important for keeping the skin healthy. Add ½ to 2 teaspoons (depending on the dog's size) of sunflower, canola, or other vegetable oil to the food every day. Your veterinarian can also give you powders, pills, or emulsions (an oily liquid) that contain zinc, biotin, and essential fatty acids.

■ **Homeopathy**
See page 79.

Susceptible breeds: Hereditary hairlessness is a characteristic of some Chihuahuas and of African, Chinese, and Mexican hairless breeds. Blue colored Dobermans, shorthaired dachshunds, whippets, and silver toy poodles often have areas where the hair falls out.

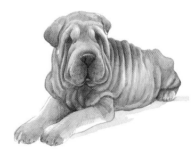

The skin folds of the Shar Pei, which are the result of selective breeding, lead to skin problems.

■ Homeopathy for Skin Disorders

The skin and fur of a dog reflect how the metabolism is working and therefore the overall state of health. Skin disorders become obvious if a dog itches excessively, the skin gets flaky, the hair becomes dull and brittle or falls out—often accompanied by eczema brought on by scratching and licking.

The homeopath regards the skin as, among other things, a detoxifying organ. In the case of many skin diseases it is therefore helpful to start out by cleansing the system.

Regimen for Internal Cleansing
• 3 days without solid food. Give only water so that the organism does not have to deal with any additional metabolic by-products;
• 4th day: 1 tablespoon of meat mixed with herbs, such as parsley, water cress, or a little garlic, and with 1 tablespoon rolled oats, rice, or bran;
• 5th day: 2 tablespoons of each;
• 6th day: 3 tablespoons of each;
• each following day 1 tablespoon more of each until the normal daily portion is reached.

Important: 1 fasting day per week. Check with your veterinarian if food deprivation is safe for your pet.

This regimen is very beneficial to the organism.

Treatment with Blood from the Organism Itself
Experienced homeopaths often successfully use this treatment for skin disorders of an allergic nature. A little blood is taken from the sick dog, diluted with the approapriate homeopathic solutions, and then injected again.

Treatment at Home
The following remedies can be used to treat the dog at home (for dosage, see page 39):
• For dry skin, tendency to develop eczema (aggravated by rainy weather), unpleasant smell, dandruff, hair loss, dull coat, excessive thirst, hard stool alternating with diarrhea: Sulfur. This leads to better blood flow to the skin especially in chronic conditions.
• For dandruff, itching, acne, puffy skin: *Calcium carbonicum.*
• For dry skin, dandruff, severe itching (especially at night and when it's hot): *Psorinum.*
• For dry, cracked skin including on the nipples and scrotum: Petroleum.
• For hair loss: Selenium. If, in females, the hair is falling out in the kidney area in a symmetrical pattern and without itching, consult the section on homeopathy under False Pregnancy, page 73.
• For nettle-like rashes, a penetrating and sour smell, itching, swellings in the head area: *Acidum formicicum, Urtica urens.*
• For brittle hair on the back above the lower ribs: *Lycopodium.* This is often a symptom of liver disease.
• For suppurating rashes: *Lachesis*, phosphorus, *Pyrogenium.*
• For eczema on the toes: *Silicea.*
• For allergic skin conditions with itching but no other changes: Sulfur, *Vincetoxicum, Natrium muriaticum.*
• For allergic reaction to grass and pollen in the spring: *Urtica urens. Acidum formicicum* can be given prophylactically before the grass flowers.

Important: For external, localized application the skin should be shaved and dabbed with a 2% hydrogen peroxide solution. Then apply ointment or oil-containing *Calendula, Arnica, Calcium carbonicum,* or *Symphytum.*

5

Bacterial Skin Disorders

Eczema is a collective term for changes in the skin caused by inflammation. Scratching and licking then lead to a purulent infection.

Symptoms: Reddened skin, small, nodular raised spots, purulent blisters, patches of oozing or bare skin.

Causes and effects:
• Acute itching caused by parasites (fleas, lice, and mites), insect bites, allergies, skin injuries. Scratching and biting can result in oozing wounds on the hips, base of tail, head, and neck.
• Abnormally deep folds in the skin develop oozing eczema (called skin fold pyoderma or interdermal dermatitis).
• Overproduction of skin oil (sebum) leads to purulent inflammation of the sebaceous glands. Short-haired puppies develop acne and boils on the head and belly; older, long-haired dogs get seborrheic eczema and folliculitis (see Glossary, page 116) primarily on the belly and back.
• Injuries and foreign bodies lodged in the skin (thorns, wood splinters, tick mouth parts) cause bloody and oozing abscesses on and between the toes (pododermatitis).

● **Treatment**
You can combat insect parasites yourself with flea baths (see page 82). Keep the dog from scratching and licking by putting an Elizabethan collar (available from your veterinarian, see drawing, page 22) on it, or covering up the sore place with a bandage or a piece of material cut to the right shape.

If these remedies don't work take the dog the veterinarian. He or she will shave the affected area to examine the kind and extent of the skin changes. This also allows the skin to dry better, and localized treatment is more effective.
• For overproduction of sebum and folliculitis medicinal baths are helpful (bath additives available from your veterinarian).
• For disinfecting sores, use a 2% hydrogen peroxide solution or dilute povidone iodine.
• Ointments and powders containing zinc are used on weeping eczema.
• Antibiotic ointments and emulsions are applied to wounds that produce a lot of pus.
• For extensive purulent eczema and abscesses, give antibiotic tablets in addition to using ointment. At the beginning, cortisone is given as well to counteract inflammation and itching.

Follow-up care: Disinfect the affected places twice a day and rub in any prescribed medication. Baths twice a week. Anti-biotic pills usually have to be given for 2 to 3 weeks. For purulent infections on the paws, soak the paws in camomile baths daily and keep them bandaged.

■ **Homeopathy**
See page 79.

Susceptible breeds:
• Skin fold pyoderma on the head occurs primarily in short-nosed breeds, such as Pekingese and pugs; in Shar Peis it tends to affect the entire body (see drawing, page 78).
• Furunculosis and dermatitis caused by biting occur primarily in German shepherds, but can affect any breed.

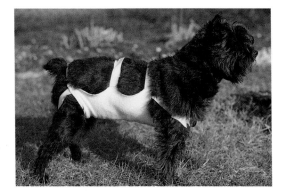

A kind of undergarment, home-made to fit the dog, is often the best protection against the dog's licking sores and wounds.

Skin Disorders Caused by Fungi (Ringworm)

Symptoms: Round, hairless spots with red ring around darkly discolored skin; sometimes the hair comes out by the handful with dandruff sticking to the base of the hairs; moderate itching made worse by scratching.

Causes and effects: Fungi such as *Microsporum* and *Trichophyton* all over the body. In skin folds and between toes, yeasts and fungi cause scaliness and oozing of the skin.

Note: Humans can pick up fungus diseases from dogs and can develop very persistent skin problems; also, dogs can "catch" fungal infections from their owners. Good hygiene is therefore important. Always wash your hands every time after handling the dog (see also Important Notes, page 127).

● **Treatment**

➡ The veterinarian will take a culture of the fungus to pinpoint the causative agent. Often the dog has to be clipped all over in order so that the extent of the infection can be evaluated.

● Treat localized infections with a disinfectant, such as povidone iodine solution, and apply an antifungal ointment twice a day. For severe and extensive infections, antimycotic drugs also have to be given orally twice a day.

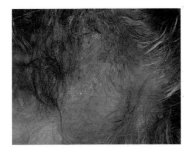

Dermatitis caused by the dog's biting itself.

● For bathing the entire coat and for disinfecting the environment (basket, blankets, sleeping spots), solutions containing imidazole (available from the veterinarian) work well.

● Vitamin and mineral supplements (available from the veterinarian or at pet stores) and the addition of polyunsaturated vegetable oil to the food improve the regenerating powers of the skin.

Follow-up care: Keep disinfecting affected areas and applying ointment to them 2 to 3 times a day and continue giving baths twice a week (wash your hands thoroughly afterwards). Have the veterinarian check the dog weekly. The fur may have to be clipped again. Sometimes antimycotic drugs (see Glossary, page 114) in tablet form have to be continued for 3 to 4 weeks.

Prevention: When you groom your dog, check for matted fur and skin changes (see page 18).

■ **Homeopathy**
See page 79.

Skin Disorders Caused by Parasites

Symptoms: Itching and eczema, especially on the head, neck, and back, but sometimes all over.

Causes: Skin parasites (fleas, biting and sucking lice; between 1.5 and 3 mm in size) can be spotted in the fur with the naked eye.

● Lice leave sticky egg masses on the hairs.

● Flea droppings (tiny black dots) contain blood and therefore leave a red area if placed on a damp tissue.

● Ticks attach themselves primarily to the head and neck and range from pin-head size to pea size when they are full of blood.

Effects: Chronic and sometimes allergic eczema from scratching, sometimes with hair loss. The dog flea is a carrier of the most common tapeworm found in dogs (*Dipylidium caninum*). Ticks transmit a bacterial joint and skin disease (Lyme disease, borelliosis), which afflicts both dogs and humans and can take a chronic form. Ticks also transmit a viral meningitis that humans are subject to but that is no threat to dogs.

● **Treatment**

● Fleas and biting and sucking lice: Wash the dog with an appropriate insecticidal

5

shampoo 2 to 3 times a week. In addition to shampoos, powders and sprays against parasites are available (from your veterinarian or from pet stores).
• At the same time, the dog's surroundings have to be disinfected with insecticides (see Glossary, page117) because fleas spend only 15 to 20 percent of the time on the dog sucking blood. In heated rooms fleas can prey on a dog all year round.
• Ticks: Dab a drop of oil on the tick, wait a minute or two, then carefully extract the tick with special tick tweezers, turning it back and forth slowly to make sure the head does not come off and stay in the skin.

Follow-up care: Continue the suggested treatment until the parasites are gone.

Prevention: Put a flea collar (available at pet stores) on the dog. The collar exudes insecticide for about 3 to 4 months.

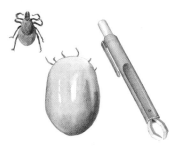

A special kind of forceps is helpful for removing ticks.

This means, however, that both humans and dog are exposed to the toxins. The collar should therefore be removed and put in an airtight bag while the dog is indoors in order to minimize exposure to the smell and insecticide.

■ Homeopathy
See page 79.

Mange

Symptoms:
• Sarcoptic mange: Severe itching; small lumps and scabs forming on head and legs and later all over. Reddening of skin, open sores, and scabby places from scratching; patches of hair loss (moth-eaten look).
• Demodectic mange: At first, light flaking, reddening of skin in hairless places, especially on head and legs. Afflicts mainly puppies. Later many small, pus-filled pimples and hairless spots with bluish red, thickened skin mostly near the eyes, lips, and ears, also on paws.

Causes and effects:
• Sarcoptic mange: An allergic reaction to the mites of *Sarcoptes canis,* and *Sarcoptes scabiei,* which makes the dog scratch and bite itself and results in large hairless patches and pus-filled lesions (pyoderma).
• Demodectic mange: The mite *Demodex canis* lives in the hair follicles of many dogs and normally causes no problems. But

A Bath against Parasites

Bathe your dog the way you wash your hair. Wet the hair, apply shampoo, and massage the skin for a good 5 to 10 minutes. Be sure also to disinfect (with an insect spray) the blankets, rugs, pillows and other places the dog likes to lie on.

if the immune system is weakened, the mites multiply rapidly and cause mange, particularly in puppies.

Note: Sarcoptic mange can be transmitted to humans.

● Treatment
➡ Because mange is contagious to humans it is essential to take the dog to the veterinarian. Sometimes dog owners don't realize their pet has mange until they notice red and very itchy bumps on their own arms.

For a precise diagnosis skin scrapings (see Glossary, page 119) are examined under the microscope for mites. It is important to clip the entire body because the mites can be anywhere. Use an insecticidal rinse once a week and allow it to develop its full effect by drying on the body. In case of major infestations, insecticides (such as Ivermectin) may also have to be given as injections or pills.

• Strain on the immune system caused by worm infestations and other infections plays a role especially in demodectic mange. Therefore, cortisone to control itching should only be administered if prescribed by a veterinarian because this drug further weakens the immune system.

Follow-up care: Insecticidal baths or rinses once a week. Apply antibiotic ointment 2 to 3 times a day to ulcerating eczema resulting from scratching. Take the dog to the veterinarian for weekly or biweekly check-ups. Treatment of demodectic mange should be considered successful only if the symptoms don't recur for 6 months.

Prevention: Check the skin when grooming your dog. Deworm regularly and keep immunization up to date (see Vaccination Schedule, page 20).

■ **Homeopathy**
See page 79.

Skin Allergy Resulting from Direct Contact

Symptoms: Itching and redness, bumpy skin, weepy spots, and crusts primarily on thinly haired places, such as the belly, the inside of the thighs, the armpits, and the anal and genital region; seen most frequently from spring to fall.

Causes: Appears within 1 to 3 days after exposure to irritants in the surroundings, such as chemicals in paints, cleansers, plants, and insecticides (if in flea collar, symptoms appear on the neck).

Effects: Licking and scratching, which result in oozing eczema.

● **Treatment**
The dog owner has to watch when symptoms appear and what kind of contact causes them. If the irritant can be determined, avoid further contact. If this is impracticable in the long run, emulsions and ointments containing cortisone have to be used.

Follow-up care: If skin irritation persists after the skin condition caused by biting and scratching (see page 80) has been treated, small doses of cortisone may have to be given, perhaps over a prolonged period.

■ **Homeopathy**
See page 79.

Susceptible breeds: Light-colored, short-haired dogs, such as yellow Labradors, boxers, and beagles.

Skin Allergy Resulting from Indirect Contact

Symptoms: Itching and redness on the head and neck, later all over. Urticaria or nettle rash (an acute allergic reaction) causes blisters and wheals up to $\frac{3}{8}$ inch (1 cm) in diameter that can develop into large swollen areas.

Causes:
• Food allergy: Ingredients (mostly in dry food) the animal is allergic to; sometimes the allergy also causes diarrhea at first.
• Inhalant allergy (atopy): In most cases a congenital overreaction of the organism to plant pollen, the spores of fungi, house dust, or dandruff and hair of other animals or people. The reaction takes the form of skin changes or, only rarely, "hay fever."
• Nettle rash is a reaction in most cases to insect bites but can also be caused by food ingredients, medications, and inhaled allergens (substances that trigger allergies).

Effects: Licking, scratching, and biting; this causes acute eczema (see page 80) with weeping places and scabs.

5

● Treatment

In case of food allergy, put the dog on an allergy diet (see page 25).

➤ The veterinarian may be able to determine the allergen through an allergy test. If the allergen is not food-related, treatment with a series of desensitizing injections (see Glossary, page 116) is often successful. If contact with the causative agent cannot be avoided over the long run, or if the allergen cannot be determined, cortisone has to be given for an extended period in as low a dosage as possible.

Follow-up care: Depending on the case, give cortisone for several weeks in the spring or a few months toward the fall since allergies often occur in the warm season only.

■ Homeopathy
See page 79.

Susceptible breeds: Boxers, Labrador retrievers, and German shepherds more than other dogs have a hereditary predisposition to inhalant allergy.

Skin Problems Caused by Autoimmune Reaction

Symptoms: Initially, blisterlike rash that breaks open and then weeps; found especially on the head and near the muzzle, nose, ears, anus, and genitals, less commonly on paws and other parts of the body. Lethargy, fever, refusal of food as in the case of an infection.

Causes: Abnormal behavior of the immune cells, which no longer recognize some of the body's own substances as such. This condition is thought to be caused by virus infections, side effects to drugs, and environmental factors, such as pollutants and ionizing or solar radiation.

Effects: Serious, chronic impairment of overall health.

● Treatment
➤ Autoimmune disorders of the skin are usually incurable. Veterinarians can prescribe cortisone to combat and alleviate the symptoms.

Follow-up care: Cortisone as needed to control symptoms but, because of the side effects, at lowest possible dosage. Cortisone treatment usually has to be continued for life. For the so-called collie nose (a der-

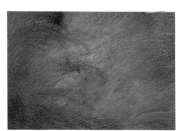

This scab formation suggests mange.

matitis on the nose caused by prolonged exposure to the sun), localized application of a cortisone ointment generally suffices, but many of these dogs may develop skin cancer on their unpigmented nose after several years.

Prevention: For collie nose, lotions with a high sunscreen factor help.

Susceptible breeds: Collies, shelties, German shepherds, and huskies tend to develop collie nose.

Skin Tumors

Lumps that can be moved with the skin; usually in the head, neck, and back areas.

Causes and Effects: Growths, most commonly of the sebaceous glands. They can grow as big as Ping-Pong balls and sometimes break open, leaving craterlike, ulcerating wounds. Usually benign; most common in old dogs.

● Treatment
➤ These masses should to be removed by the veterinarian, especially if they keep refilling after draining. All tumors should be surgically removed and subjected to laboratory analysis to establish whether they are malignant.

Follow-up treatment: Clean the incision twice daily. The stitches should be removed after 10 days.

Susceptible breeds: Particularly in boxers skin tumors may be malignant.

Hormone-induced Disorders

Here only those hormonal problems that are most common and whose symptoms are relatively easy to recognize by the dog owner are discussed. A dull coat and significant, symmetrical hair loss without itching are always a clear sign of hormonal malfunctioning.

Thyroid Deficiency

Symptoms: Symmetrical hair loss with darkening of the skin (pigmentation) on the flanks, base of the tail, thighs, and back of the nose; excessive flakiness of skin and overproduction of sebum. The skin feels cool, spongy, and dry. Lethargy, fatigue, below-normal temperature, increased appetite, obesity, and lack of energy.

Causes: Congenital condition or inflammations, injuries, and tumorous growths, dietary deficiency of iodine.

Effects: Congenital thyroid deficiency results in stunted and crippled growth; dogs die prematurely.

● Treatment

➡ The veterinarian relies on special blood tests for diagnosis. Hormone tablets to be

Enlarged Thyroid Gland

The thyroid is a gland with two lobes placed, as in humans, in the laryngeal area of the throat.

The common name of an enlarged thyroid is goiter. The condition is caused either by an iodine deficiency (now rare because iodine is added to table salt and to drinking water) or by inadequate output of thyroid hormones. Giving the dog iodine or thyroid hormones quickly results in reduction and normalization of the gland.

given daily in the food are prescribed for thyroid deficiency.

Follow-up care: At first weekly visits to the veterinarian to establish the appropriate hormone dosage; later, check-ups every 3 months. Your dog will respond after just a few days, becoming more active and beginning to slim down. The hair grows back after 8 to 12 weeks. Usually thyroid hormones have to be given for life.

■ Homeopathy

For dosage, see page 39.
Jodum and *Spongia.*

Susceptible breeds: Older dogs of large breeds, such as boxers,

Dobermans, beagles, and golden retrievers.

Hyperthyroidism

Symptoms: Weight loss, increased thirst, restlessness, bulging eyes, excitabiliy, frequent panting, trembling muscles, increased pulse rate, slightly elevated body temperature, seeking out of cool spots; primarily in old dogs.

Causes: Speeding up of the metabolism because of overproduction of thyroid hormones, usually associated with thyroid cancer.

Effects: Thyroid tumors are quite rare in dogs, but, being malignant, they tend to metastasize.

● Treatment

The thyroid gland is as a rule enlarged on one side, and one can usually feel small lumps.
➡ The veterinarian will take a radiograph of the lungs to see if the cancer has already metastasized. If not, the side of the gland that is cancerous along with the lymph node next to it is surgically removed. The symptoms of hyperthyroidism are a warning sign that cancer may be developing.

■ Homeopathy

For dosage, see page 39.
Glonoinum, Acidum arsenicum.
• If weight loss: *China.*

Susceptible breeds: Boxers, golden retrievers, beagles; however, any breed can be affected.

Hyperfunction of the Adrenal Cortex

Symptoms: Symmetrical hair loss up to complete nakedness of the body (hair remains on legs and head); paper thin, darkly pigmented skin with many wrinkles and infected hair pores (folliculitis); increased thirst and urine output; increased appetite; obesity; potbelly (see drawing) caused by enlarged liver; lethargy, muscle weakness, trembling, below-normal temperature.

Causes: Overproduction of hormones by the adrenal cortex (Cushing's syndrome). The cortex of the adrenal glands, which are located in the fatty tissues of the kidneys, produces among other hormones a form of cortisone called cortisol. Usually overproduction of the hormone is due to a malfunctioning of the pituitary gland (hypophysis), which plays a central role in the regulation of hormone production. Rarely, the condition is caused by tumors on the adrenal cortex.

Effects: Ulcerating infection of the skin, of internal organs, and throughout the organism, caused by the elevated cortisol level, which lowers the body's resistance to pathogens and physical stress.

● **Treatment**
➡ The veterinarian uses special tests of the hormone levels in the blood to arrive at a diagnosis. Most growths on the adrenal glands, respond to a treatment with one or more cytostatic drugs (see Chemotherapeutic, Glossary, page 115) that slows down cortisol production in the adrenal cortex. Correct dosage has to be carefully established and checked daily at first. Small tumors on the adrenal glands can sometimes be surgically removed.

Follow-up care: Treatment has to continue for life. The dog's thirst has to be watched and controlled for the first week. For maintenance treatment, one dose a week usually suffices. Regular checks by the veterinarian every 3 to 4 months are necessary. After 6 to 8 weeks the hair will begin to grow back, and after 3 to 4 months the dog will look normal again.

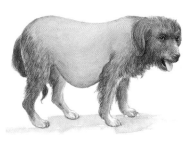

Cushing's syndrome: Hanging potbelly and hair loss.

Insufficiency of the Adrenal Cortex

Symptoms: Listlessness, poor appetite, weight loss, fatigue, general weakness, vomiting, diarrhea, and circulatory problems with irregular pulse, staggering, collapse.

Causes: The activity of the adrenal cortex may be impaired by injury sustained in an accident, by infections, tumors, or insufficient blood flow. Stressful situations or the sudden discontinuance of prolonged cortisone therapy can also lead to insufficiency of the adrenal cortex (Addison's disease).

Effects: Serious decline in general health and acute circulatory problems that can lead to shock and sudden death.

● **Treatment**
➡ A special hormone test is used to diagnose this condition. Acute circulatory problems are treated with intravenous injections to which the lacking hormones are at first added.

Follow-up care: When the dog comes home from the animal clinic it is given hormones in tablet form twice a day or as injections every 10 days. Usually hormone treatments are necessary for life.

Prevention: Avoid stressful situations, excitement, and excessive exertion.

Diabetes

Symptoms: Excessive thirst and frequent urinating, listlessness, lethargy, voracious appetite without weight gain, and, in the final stage, weight loss; dull coat; occasionally itching; pot-belly because of enlarged liver, breath odor resembling acetone; cataracts. Diabetes affects primarily older dogs.

Causes: Diabetes is caused by inadequate insulin (a hormone that is produced in the pancreas and regulates the metabolism of sugar).

Effects: Because of the lack of insulin the blood sugar rises to many times the normal level. This upsets the entire metabolism, leading to heart, kidney, liver, and eye problems and eventually to death.

● **Treatment**
You can check your dog's urine for sugar quite easily with a test strip (available from drug stores). Normal urine does not contain sugar.
➤ To diagnose the problem more accurately, the veterinarian takes a blood sample. Depending on the blood sugar level, insulin therapy with daily injections is initiated. It may be better to keep the dog under supervision in the animal clinic for 3 to 5 days since 2 to 3 daily blood sugar tests are necessary to establish the proper insulin dosage. After these ini-

tial days blood sugar checks should be done weekly at first, then monthy, and later perhaps every 3 months.
Just as important as the insulin injections is a strict and consistent diet with 3 to 4 feedings given in the course of the day. (see Diet for Diabetes, page 25). The insulin injections should be given every day at the same time, about 4 to 6 hours before the first feeding (see Insulin Injections, page 23).

Follow-up care: The dog has to stay on a diabetic diet and get insulin shots for life. It always has to have plenty of drinking water available. By watching how much the dog drinks and occasionally checking the sugar in the urine with a test strip, the insulin dosage can be finely adjusted. If the dog is clearly drinking more than usual, the dosage should be increased slightly; if it drinks less, the dosage is slightly lowered. A dog can live quite comfortably for many years if it is given a proper diet and insulin shots.

■ **Homeopathy**
For dosage, see page 39.
Syzygium jambolanum, Aesculus, Phlorizinum, Plumbum metallicum. However, this potentially fatal disorder demands a conventional veterinarian treatment first.

Susceptible breeds: Diabetes is found most often in medium-

sized dogs, such as poodles, dachshunds, Pomeranians, and fox, Welsh, and hunting terriers, but it can occur in all breeds and mongrels.

The Crucial Bit of Sugar

If an overdose of insulin is given or if the dog doesn't eat after an insulin injection, the blood sugar level may drop below normal. This can be fatal. Signs are nervousness, trembling, tiredness, staggering, cramping, and loss of consciousness.
Give your dog some sugar as quickly as possible. The best way is to dribble sugar water into the mouth or to smear some honey or karo syrup or corn syrup on the tongue. You should always carry a cube of sugar with you on walks with a diabetic dog in case of an emergency. You can also take the dog to the veterinarian, who will, depending on the blood sugar level, inject a variably concentrated glucose solution into the veins.

5

Disorders of the Musculoskeletal and Nervous Systems

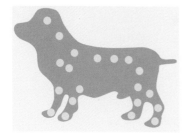

*D*ogs, like most vertebrate animals, have a flexible spine. At one end is the head and at the other, the tail. The front legs are supported by the spine at the shoulders via muscles; the back legs, at the pelvis by a more solid bone-to-bone connection. The skeleton supports the body and gives it its external shape. The rigid skeletal system is made flexible through the joints. But it is the muscles that enable a dog to run, jump, and sit.

The bone growth in a puppy happens primarily in the cartilagenous layers at the upper and lower ends of the long bones and on the skull and pelvis. Congenital bone diseases, an incorrect and usually overly rich diet, and damage to the cartilagenous bone connections can result in painful malformations in bones and joints that cause various forms of lameness.

Hip Dysplasia

Symptoms: Dogs seem somewhat lazy because of the disability; they may be lame in one or both rear legs and have difficulty getting up and lying down; they have a swinging or waddling gait and are often knock-kneed.

Causes and effects: Canine hip dysplasia (CHD) is in most cases due to a hereditary bone deformity that afflicts mostly large, heavy dogs. It is exacerbated by diet and excessive activity in predisposed breeds. During the period of growth, the head or "ball" of the femur develops a shape that doesn't quite fit the pelvic cup (see picture of X-ray, following page). Use and increasing weight cause abnormal wear, and premature osteoarthritis develops in the hip joints. The dogs become lame and can move only with great pain.

● Treatment
➡ Hip dysplasia can be diagnosed only with the help of pelvic radiographs. It is treated with anti-inflammatory pain medication. For acute problems resulting from too much strain on or added injury to the joint, cortisone has to be given as well for a few days, preferably in tablet form.

In dogs that are still growing, a relatively minor operation in which a muscle on the inside of the thigh is severed helps relieve pain.

If the pain is severe and constant, hip replacement has become the standard treatment. This operation is expensive and performed only in special clinics, but it can work wonders. Just one day after the operation, the dogs can put some weight on the back legs again, and a week or two later they walk without apparent pain. An alternative to this expensive operation is excisional arthroplasty, in which the head of the femur is removed. This alleviates the pain, but in heavy breed dogs does not provide quite as satisfactory a solution as full hip replacement.

Follow-up treatment: Anti-inflammatory pain medication is given for 4 to 8 days in decreasing doses. Depending on the severity of the condition, the pain killers, combined with cortisone if indicated, can be resorted to repeatedly, but always wait at least 3 to 4 weeks before using them again.

Important: All pain killers may produce side effects (damage of the bone marrow, anemia) if used over long periods, and should only be used in consultation with your veterinarian. Cortisone, too, should be used only if absolutely necessary and not given on a permanent basis because it lowers the body's resistance.

Prevention: Don't give growing dogs overly rich food because this seems to encourage the development of hip dysplasia. Exclude dogs with this disorder from breeding.

Susceptible breeds: CHD is the most widespread hereditary canine disease. It occurs in almost all breeds, though with greater frequency in large, heavy dogs, such as German shepherds, Great Danes, Saint Bernards, mastiffs, bulldogs, Bernese mountain dogs, and sheep dogs. Nearly all breeders' associations of large as well as medium-sized dogs now require that pelvic radiographs be taken when the dogs are 18 months to 2 years old. The result determines whether or not the dog is considered fit for breeding.

Necrosis of the Ball of the Hip

Symptoms: Dogs between 5 and 10 months of age develop lameness in one hindleg.

Causes and effects: In small breeds, such as Yorkshire terriers and poodles, a congenital deformity of the head of the femur (presumably caused by impaired blood supply) results in necrosis of the upper half of the ball in the hip joint.

● Treatment
➡ An exact diagnosis is based on radiographs. The only possible treatment is surgical removal of the head of the femur (excision arthroplsty). The connective tissue between the pelvis and the femur forms a substitute joint.

Follow-up care: Usual postoperative care of the incision (see pages 22 and 23) and removal of the sutures after 10 days. The dogs begin to put some weight on the operated leg after a few days, but it can be weeks before the lameness disappears. Afterwards the dogs usually move without problems for the rest of their lives.

Prevention: Dogs with this condition should be excluded from breeding. The desire of breeders to produce ever smaller dogs is one of the factors contributing to deformities such as this and slipping kneecaps (see page 90).

Susceptible breeds: This congenital abnormality occurs only in small breeds, such as Yorkshire terriers, Chihuahuas, Maltese, Shih Tzus, and toy versions of poodles, schnauzers, and pinschers.

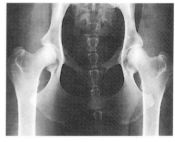

X-ray of a healthy hip joint: The ball part of the femur fits snugly into the pelvic socket.

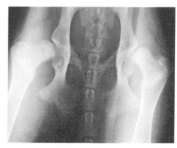

X-ray of the same joint in a dog with hip dysplasia: The ball part and the socket no longer fit together properly.

Slipping Kneecap (Luxating Patella)

Symptoms: At first, hopping, then frequent lifting of one or both hindlegs. Thickening, painful stifle joint (the canine counterpart of the human knee). If both legs are affected, the dog hops with rounded back like a rabbit. The first symptoms show up at 4 to 6 months.

Causes and Effects: Congenital deformity of the hindlegs. Because of a twisting and bending of the femur, the kneecap (patella) slips out of its normal place and inward (medial patellar dislocation). Abnormal wear then causes arthritis and stiffening of the joint.

● Treatment
➡ There are several surgical procedures to correct patellar dislocation. Your veterinarian can explain them to you.

Follow-up treatment: Follow the usual rules for treating the wound after surgery (see pages 22 and 23). Keep the dog from overexerting and walk it on the leash for 3 to 4 weeks. For a week or two after surgery the dogs are more reluctant to put weight on the joints, but after that they improve steadily.

Prevention: Affected dogs should not be used for breeding.

Susceptible breeds: Primarily small dogs, such as Yorkshire terriers, Chihuahuas, Shih Tzus, and toy versions of poodles, schnauzers, and pinschers.

Hypertrophic Osteodystrophy

Symptoms: Increased bone volume at the carpal, hock, or stifle joint, which feels warm to the touch and is painful. Lameness, fever, apathy, poor appetite.

Causes and effects: In large, rapidly growing breeds, puppies 3 to 6 months old develop excess bone tissue if they are fed a diet too high in proteins and calories. Overdosing with vitamins has also been suggested as a cause. The excess growth occurs on the long leg bones near the wrist, hock, and sometimes the stifle and results in deformed joints.

● Treatment
➡ The veterinarian uses X-rays to diagnose the condition. Analgesic drugs (see Glossary, page 114) are effective against pain and fever. The most important measure, though, is to change to a diet higher in fiber. Reduce regular meat and replace it with high quality commercial dog food, and mix more fibrous carbohydrates, such as vegetables and whole grains into the food. Reduce the amount of food, and omit supplements. When growth is completed, the disease disappears, but the bone deformities remain.

On the Topic of Rickets

Dogs are often overfed vitamins because dog owners, breeders, and sometimes, unfortunately, even veterinarians think that this will eliminate the danger of rickets. However, rickets (caused by vitamin D deficiency) is very seldom a problem for dogs in our latitudes, and it has in fact practically disappeared because just about all commercial dog food is fortified with vitamins. On the other hand, a diet based too much on meat can lead to osteoporosis, which is caused by the low calcium and high phosphorus content of animal proteins (meat as well as milk products). Osteoporosis has nothing to do with rickets and can easily be corrected with calcium supplements.

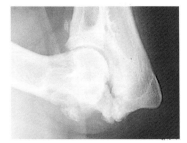

Arthritis in the elbow: Wear and tear gradually cause painful changes of the joint.

Elbow Dysplasia and Osteochondritis

Symptoms:
• Elbow dysplasia: Lameness in one or both front legs, especially noticeable after the dog has been lying down or walking downhill for some time.
• Osteochondritis: Pain and lameness caused by damage to the cartilage in the shoulder, elbow, stifle, and hock joints.
   Both disorders develop in large dogs 6 to 8 months old.
   Causes and effects:
• Elbow dysplasia: Uneven lengthening of the ulna and radius (see drawing of skeleton, page 34), which results from injuries to the growing ends of the long bones. The uneven length of the bones leads to improper distribution of weight, faulty union of one of the elbow bones (anconeal process, see Glossary, page 114) and, later, to arthritis.
• Osteochondritis: Separation of joint cartilage, pieces of which float freely in the joint, causing lameness and, later, chronic arthritis.
   Both disorders are more likely to develop if there is stress on the joints or if the puppy's diet is too rich.

● **Treatment**
➡ Surgery undertaken at an early enough stage keeps arthritis at a minimal level.
   Follow-up care: The usual postoperative care of the inci-

sion (see pages 22 and 23) and removal of sutures after 10 days. Keep the dog from over-exerting and walk it mostly on the leash for 3 to 4 weeks. If arthritis develops, it requires lifelong treatment. Surgery does not correct the primary problem but merely slows the arthritic process.
   Prevention: Exclude dogs with these conditions from breeding.

Susceptible breeds: Big, large-boned dogs, such as Great Danes, German shepherds, Saint Bernards, basset hounds, Bernese mountain dogs, boxers, golden retrievers, Weimaraners, pointers, German wirehaired pointers. Elbow dysplasia also occurs in dachshunds.

Bone Infection (Osteomyelitis)

Symptoms: High fever, swelling, noticeable warmth

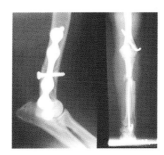

Stabilization of a broken bone with a pin and bone screw.

and obvious painfulness in the area of the affected bone, oozing wounds that keep breaking open, extreme lameness.
   Causes: Infectious inflammation of the bone and the bone marrow following open fractures or faulty bone growth. The infected bone literally disintegrates, and hollow spaces form from which pus drains through a sinus tract connecting the bone to the skin.

● **Treatment**
➡ High doses of antibiotics are necessary and surgery may be required.
   Follow-up care: Only continued high doses of antibiotics for several weeks are likely to help.

Susceptible breeds: German shepherd puppies between 5 and 12 months of age sometimes develop painful inflammations without infection on the humerus or the femur (panosteitis). This condition, which is sometimes called "growing pains," is characterized by fever and by lameness that shifts from one leg to another. This is apparently an autoimmune reaction (see page 95) and usually disappears again spontaneously after 1 to 3 months. Pain medication helps control the discomfort.

6

Arthritis

Symptoms: Variable to very severe lameness; increased warmth and thickening of the affected joint or joints. Fever, apathy, lack of appetite.

Causes and effects: Infection of joints that is caused generally by injuries but can also be introduced by bacteria carried into the joint in the blood. The infection causes destruction of the joint cartilage and stiffening of the joints. Rheumatoid arthritis occurs in dogs and is a result of autoimmune reactions (see page 95).

● **Treatment**

➡ The veterinarian diagnoses the condition on the basis of radiographs. Surgical opening and drainage of the affected joint, disinfectant irrigation, antibiotics, and analgesic drugs.

• Rheumatoid arthritis is treated with anti-inflammatory analgesics. Cortisone therapy usually brings noticeable improvement.

Follow-up care: The veterinarian irrigates the joint over a period of 3 to 5 days. Anti-inflammatory, analgesic, and antibiotic drugs may be continued for several weeks. If there is an congenital tendency to rheumatoid arthritis, the drugs may have to be continued for life.

Prevention: Consult the veterinarian for even the most minor joint injuries.

■ Homeopathy for Chronic Arthritis

A veterinarian schooled in homeopathy regards the dog's manifestation of pain—limping—as a sign that the affected joint should receive less strain and stress. If the pain is suppressed with "pain killers," so that the animal can put weight on the hurting foot again, this will in time cause further damage to the tissue. Don't be afraid to let the dog limp for a while but see to it that weight is put on the hurting leg as little as possible. Homeopathic remedies can not only prevent further deterioration but also achieve significant improvement.

Basic Treatment
For dosage, see page 39.
• For dogs up to 6 years old: *Traumeel.*
• For older dogs: *Zeel.*

Further Remedies
For dosage, see page 39.
• Shoulder joint: *Ferrum metallicum, Ferrum phosphoricum, Spirea ulmaria.*
• Elbow joint: *Ferrum metallicum, Colocynthis, Causticum, Hekla lava, Rhus toxicodendron, Mercurius praecipatus ruber.*
• Hip joint: Graphites (for heavy dogs); *Calcium carbonicum, Rhus toxicodendron, Pyrogenium,* and *Bryonia* (if hips hurt badly even when dog is not moving); *Lithium carbonicum, Natrium carbonicum,* and *Colchicum* (if the dog hardly feels pain even when moving but a crunching sound like snow underfoot is heard in the joint; this is due to a lack of lubricant in the joint, and the dog is especially lame during changes in the weather).
• Knee joint: *Asafoetida,* graphites, *Bryonia, Rhus toxicodendron, Kalmia, Calcium carbonicum.*

Chronic Arthritis

Symptoms: Lameness in the affected legs, especially after the dog has been lying down for some time. The condition seems to improve with movement but recurs and is aggravated after overexertion.

Causes: Acute arthritis, too much or faulty weight bearing, congenital deformities (such as hip dysplasia, see page 88), or loose cartilage fragments in the joint (see page 91). But normal wear and tear over a lifetime also results in damage to the joints and, eventually, in chronic arthritis.

● **Treatment**

➡ The veterinarian arrives at a precise diagnosis by taking radiographs. Anti-inflammatory pain medication together with prolonged cortisone treatments controls acute discomfort. For extremely painful, chronic problems with loose cartilage fragments in the joint, the veterinarian has to resort to surgical removal of the loose matter and to irrigation of the joint. The pain of joints that can hardly move anymore can be eliminated by an operation that immobilizes the joint. The leg can still be used because the other joints bend.

Follow-up care: See Hip Dysplasia, page 88.

Prevention: Moderate but regular exercise. It's better to take the dog on four 15-minute walks than on one hour-long walk without a break. Avoid wild racing around, ball playing, or stick throwing, but still keep the dog from becoming obese. Don't let the dog sleep in a cold place or on a hard floor. At any sign of problems, expose the joint to a heat lamp. If the pain is severe, the veterinarian may use diathermy. Dogs with chronic arthritis and those with congenital joint deformities should not be bred.

Bone Tumors

Symptoms: Painful swelling on the bone and obvious limp in the affected leg. Tumors on the spinal column display the same symptoms as herniated discs (see page 94).

Causes and effects: Most bone tumors are malignant and have a tendency to spread throughout the body. As in humans, the reason for the appearance of cancerous tumors is unknown. These tumors occur primarily in large dog breeds and, unfortunately, the prognosis is not very good.

● **Treatment**

➡ Diagnosis is based on radiographs. The affected bone should be removed in its entirety as soon as possible. Even if surgery is initiated early, however, bone tumors often metastasize (see Glossary, page 118), so you should think twice before deciding to operate since surgery sometimes seems to activate metastasis. Whether or not the suffering of a dog with bone cancer should be cut short depends largely on how much enjoyment life still holds for the animal in spite of the pain.

Susceptible breeds: Bone cancer afflicts primarily dogs of large breeds, such as Great Danes, Dobermans, Bernese mountain dogs, Rottweilers, boxers, and German shepherds.

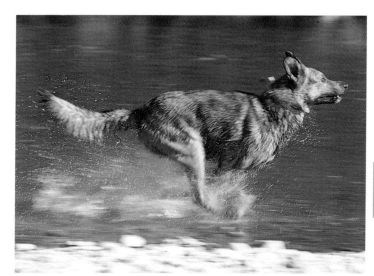

6

A well-balanced diet is very important for keeping a dog healthy.

Herniated Disc

Symptoms:
• In minor ruptures (discopathy): Refusal to climb stairs and inability to jump up into an armchair; cries of pain when being picked up, tense, arched back, stiff-legged gait, lameness, buckling of one or both front legs, tense, unnaturally outstretched neck.
• In severe ruptures (prolapsed disc): After a yelp of pain the dog's hindquarters are suddenly paralyzed (legs are stiff and cramped at first, then turn limp); if the herniated disc is in the neck, there is rigid paralysis in the front and limpness in the back.

Causes: A hereditary predisposition of so-called chondrodystrophic breeds, which causes the cartilagenous tissue of the spinal discs to become brittle any time after age 5. Or a result of the aging process after age 10. Rarely brought on by accidents or other injury.

● **Treatment**
➡ In an acute case, take the dog to the veterinarian immediately. Carry the dog in a basket or on a flat, hard surface (a board or tray) so that the spine is not subjected to movement. By taking radiographs, perhaps with injection of a contrast medium into the spinal canal, the veterinarian is able to determine the location and

■ **Homeopathy for Herniated Discs**

For dosage, see page 39.
• If sudden, shooting pain (the dog arches its back like a cat): *Colocynthis.*
• If abdomen is tensely tightened (dog pulls the tail between the legs and is extremely sensitive to touch): *Nux vomica* and *belladonna,* given hourly.
• Sudden attacks of pain in cold and damp weather: *Rhus toxicodendron.*
• Pain in the neck region, head shaking (dog hangs its head, front legs buckle): *Gelsemium, Colocynthis.*

extent of the rupture. Anti-inflammatory pain medication along with cortisone is administered. If a disc is completely prolapsed, surgery is necessary immediately.

Follow-up care: Anti-inflammatory pain medication for 4 to 6 days. Exposure to heat lamp twice a day for 15 minutes (if the dog is at home). Keep the dog absolutely still, perhaps with the help of sedatives. Take it out only when it has to relieve itself, and carry it up and down stairs.

Prevention: Carry a dog with disc problems on stairs, especially when descending. Keep it from jumping off things like the sofa and from wild playing.

Susceptible breeds: Long-backed and short-legged breeds, such as dachshunds, bassets, and Welsh corgies; also poodles, Pekingese, spaniels, and schnauzers.

Ossification of the Spine (Spondylosis)

Symptoms: At first, arched back, difficulty getting up, stiff-legged gait, painful response to touch in the loin region. In advanced stages, weakness of the hindquarters but with little pain, dragging feet when walking (the middle nails are worn down), wasting of muscles.

Causes: Excessive mobility of the vertebrae because of "loose" discs; sometimes due to chronic infections, over dosage of Vitamin A.

Effects: Ossification of the spine (spondylosis). The hindlegs grow weak, and the dog becomes almost unable to get up anymore.

● **Treatment**
➡ Diagnosis is based on radiographs. Anti-inflammatory pain medication; if severe discomfort, cortisone for 3 to 4 days. Exposure to heat lamp to relax tense muscles.

Follow-up care, prevention: Rest, restricted movement. Avoid strain on the back as well as dampness and cold.

■ Homeopathy

For dosage, see page 39.
Colocynthis, Zeel.

Susceptible breeds: Most common in boxers.

Autoimmune Disorders of the Muscles; Myasthenia Gravis

Symptoms: Cramping and swelling of the muscles in the head together with prolapsed third eyelid and fever. Animal tires quickly. Stiff, awkward gait, muscle tremors, collapse after minor exertion.

Causes: Autoimmune processes that cause recurrent inflammation of the muscles (myositis) in the head region occur primarily in young German shepherds. Older dogs of this breed are sometimes subject to a general muscle weakness caused by malfunctioning transmission of impulses between nerves and muscles (myasthenia).

● Treatment

➡ The animal has to be taken to the veterinarian for diagnosis and treatment. The veterinarian will prescribe medication to relax the muscles and cortisone for the autoimmune disorder.

Follow-up care: Cortisone therapy continued over a prolonged period, first in high doses, then tapering to as low a maintenance dosage as possible, which the dog may have to stay on for life.

Prevention: Exclude affected animals from breeding, since a predisposition to this disorder is apparently hereditary.

Susceptible breeds: Both forms of the disorder occur primarily in German shepherds.

Epilepsy

Symptoms: Falling over, collapsing, convulsive trembling with stiffly extended legs and head stretched upward, compulsive chewing motions and foaming at the mouth, legs going through running motions while dog is lying down, dilated pupils, loss of consciousness, tongue turning blue because of temporarily stopped breathing.

Causes: Convulsions due to brain damage resulting from inflammations, injury with brain hemorrhage, or tumors. Epilectic seizures can also be partially or entirely due to insufficient blood flow to the brain (because of heart disease, see page 59), low blood sugar (because of diabetes, see page 87), hormonal activity (estrogen during estrus), or severe kidney or liver damage (see page 50) after contact with various kinds of poison (such as strychnine and insecticides).

● Treatment

Since in the early stages seizures usually last no more than a minute or two and are over before you have a chance even to call the veterinarian, you should concentrate on calming the dog and making sure it doesn't hurt itself.

➡ After the attack has passed, take the dog to the veterinarian. If the dog suffers from ongoing epileptic convulsions, which is rare, tranquilizers or sedatives can be injected to suppress the attack.

Follow-up care: Extended treatment (for weeks or months) is necessary, with anti-epileptic pills given twice a day to suppress seizure attacks. At the same time the primary disorder, such as heart disease, is treated. Usually the dog has to stay on medication for the rest of its life.

Note: Anti-epileptic drugs are powerful sedatives that make the dog feel tired and also make it thirstier and hungrier.

Prevention: Avoid overexertion and overexcitement. Even the boundless joy and leaping about with which your dog greets you may trigger an attack.

■ Homeopathy

Don't try to experiment with homeopathic remedies. Wrong use of these remedies has sometimes aggravated seizures.

Susceptible breeds: Epileptic fits affect schnauzers, poodles, and dachshunds more than other dogs.

6

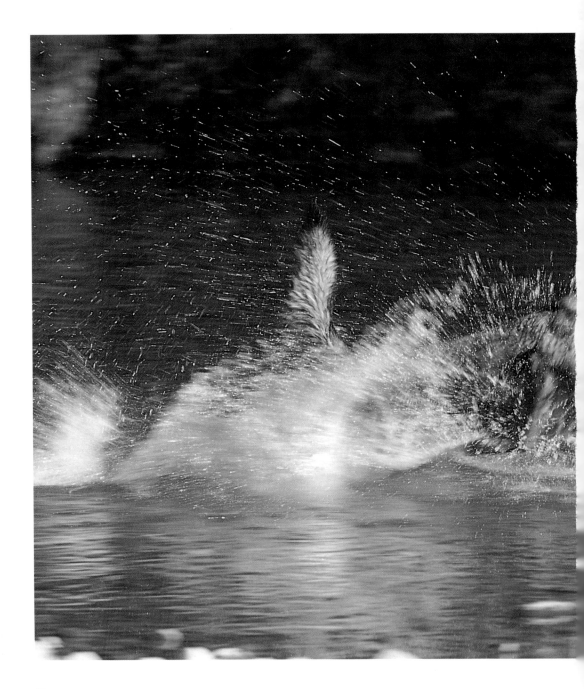

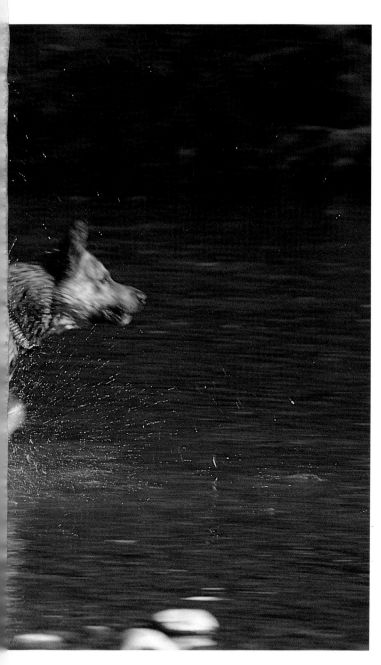

*M*ost dogs are not afraid of water. In fact, they love to get wet and even dive after thrown objects. Swimming helps keep the coat clean. Even a daily swim does no harm. The water often doesn't penetrate to the skin because the oil secreted by the skin glands makes the fur water repellant. Some dogs enter the water even in the winter. But dogs need enough exercise after getting wet for their coat to dry again; otherwise, they may become chilled.

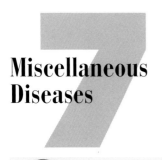

Miscellaneous Diseases

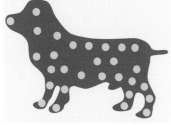

*D*ogs are susceptible to a number of infectious diseases while they are still puppies. In addition, roundworms are commonly passed on to puppies by their mother, and there are other parasites that threaten a dog's health. If you take your dog with you to a tropical country, it may bring back some tropical disease. And especially in inbred dogs of fashionable breeds, disorders typical of the breed in question may show up.

Infectious Diseases

Infectious diseases are caused by specific pathogens (viruses, bacteria, protozoans, see Glossary, page 118). They affect various organs of the body and, if left untreated, are usually fatal. However, there are highly effective vaccines available, and it is crucial that you have your puppy immunized at the proper time (see Vaccination Schedule, page 20). In the following pages the most important infectious diseases are discussed with primary emphasis on the symptoms and the typical course the disease takes since there are only very few possible treatments.

Distemper

Distemper is an extremely contagious virus infection accompanied by high fever. It occurs worldwide and can attack dogs of all ages though it is most common in puppies.

Course of the disease: Fever comes in two stages. At the beginning a high fever (as high as 105.8°F or 41°C) lasts for 24 to 48 hours. Then the temperature returns to normal (about 102°F or 39°C). The dog is apathetic, suffers from poor appetite, diarrhea, and severe conjunctivitis. The disease often goes unrecognized at this stage. After a period of from 4 to 7 days, during which the animal seems on the road to recovery, there is a secondary bacterial infection accompanied by a second bout of fever. This is followed by vomiting and diarrhea, constant coughing, and a muco-purulent discharge from eyes and nose. Almost simultaneously the dog develops gastroenteritis and pneumonia. A couple of weeks later meningitis may develop. This form of distemper, which involves the brain and brings with it further problems in the form of seizures, muscle spasms, and staggering, is incurable, and a dog that shows these symptoms should be put to sleep (see page 113).

Treatment: The veterinarian may be able to help, but only at an early stage, by injecting an immune serum. Puppies that survive distemper may not form tooth enamel properly. When the baby teeth are replaced at about 14 weeks, instead of normal, healthy teeth mere discolored stumps may grow in (so-called "distemper teeth").

Infectious Canine Hepatitis

This is a highly infectious virus infection of the liver with worldwide distribution.

Course of the disease: In its acute form, the infection comes on suddenly with a high fever. The dog grows apathetic, and dies within a few hours. In the milder form, there are 2 bouts of fever, as in the case of distemper, accompanied by similar symptoms. Pneumonia together with acute gastroenteritis visibly weakens the organism further. Typical symptoms are spontaneous bleeding in the mouth and eyes. As a result the cornea is clouded over with a milky opaqueness (blue eye). Because the liver swells up, the upper abdomen often grows big and taut and is painful when touched.

Treatment: Immune serum and antibiotics; the disease is, however, almost always fatal.

Canine Parvovirus

A contagious virus infection that appeared suddenly in the early 1980s and spread to dogs of all ages, though it most frequently attacks puppies (6 weeks to 6 months old).

Course of the disease: Constant vomiting; foamy, foul-smelling diarrhea that is frequently mixed with bright red blood; dehydration; high fever alternating with below-normal temperature; trembling, apathy; little or no appetite; abdominal pain and rumbling intestines. Essentially, the dog is suffering from enteritis, in which the mucous lining of the small intestine is damaged. Puppies that contract the disease at 4 to 10 weeks can die within a day or two from shock and heart failure. In severe cases, the disease lasts 1 to 2 weeks. A dog that survives the first week is usually out of danger.

Treatment: Immune sera somewhat reinforce the body's resistance. Initially, intravenous fluid replacement with added medication to control vomiting is essential to keep the dog alive. After 2 days of no food, a carefully supervised and gradually introduced diet (see Gastrointestinal Diet, page 24) is crucial for recovery. At the same time antibiotics are given, as well as medication to relax the intestines, counteract diarrhea, and reduce vomiting. Thorough disinfecting of the dog's surroundings is essential.

Rabies

A virus disease that also poses a threat to humans. All cases have to be reported to health authorities.

Course of the disease: Rabies is almost always transmitted through the bite of a rabid animal (the virus is in the saliva) and is generally fatal. The virus attacks the nerve tissue and ultimately culminates in encephalitis. The incubation period is about 2 weeks, but as much as a year can pass between exposure to the virus and outbreak of the disease.

The normal course is:
• Changes in behavior (lasting from a few hours to 3 days). The dog is moody, timid, restless, barks or bites without provocation, and scratches the place where the virus entered (bite wound).

• The "furious form" (1 to 4 days) is characterized by increasing restlessness and aggressiveness, chewing and destroying of objects, loss of appetite, drooling, inability to drink, prolonged howling, staggering gait, epileptic fits.
• Depression and growing exhaustion along with paralysis; death after 3 to 4 days.

Instead of the "furious form," there can be a "quiet" form, characterized by an absent gaze out of eyes with unevenly dilated pupils and by a drooping lower jaw and drooling. Death follows after 2 to 4 days.

Treatment: None. If there is any reason to suspect rabies, unvaccinated dogs are quarantined for observation and then destroyed. Specialized tests are performed on the brain and salivary gland tissues.

Leptospirosis

A disease caused by bacteria called spirochetes (genus *Leptospira*) and transmitted primarily by mice and rats. It is contagious to humans.

Course of the disease: Vomiting, diarrhea, excessive drinking, jaundice, malfunctionings of the central nervous system, coughing, and shortness of breath. The disease may affect the kidneys, liver, gastrointestinal tract, lungs, heart, brain, or eyes.

Treatment: Mild cases are curable because antibiotic drugs are relatively effective against the pathogen.

7

Kennel Cough

A respiratory disease of dogs caused by a number of viruses, and at least one species of bacteria.

Course of the disease: Coughing fits accompanied by spitting noises (suggesting inflammation of the throat and the larynx), nasal discharge, conjunctivitis, and hoarse barking. Dogs often develop kennel cough after having spent time in a shelter or kennel. The disease occurs mostly in the spring and fall.

Treatment: The urge to cough is alleviated with medication containing codeine, and mucus is reduced with decongestants (see Glossary, page 116). Antibiotics can prevent dangerous complications involving the lungs. The cough usually subsides after 1 to 2 weeks.

Tuberculosis

Rare in dogs, who can catch the disease from humans. There is no vaccine for dogs.

Course of the disease: Bouts of fever, shortness of breath, tiredness, lack of appetite, a deep, racking cough, weight loss. At a more advanced state, vomiting, diarrhea, and jaundice. The bacillus can attack all organs but most often locates in the lungs and intestines.

Treatment: Costly. Expensive medications have to be given for as long as a year or more. Danger of infection is ever present. If a case of TB has been established, all the members of the household must undergo medical examination.

Salmonellosis

Infection caused by bacteria. There is no vaccine against this disease for dogs.

Course of the disease: Simultaneous vomiting and diarrhea, sometimes with blood in the stool, apathy, fever, dehydration, general weakness. Dogs get salmonellosis mostly by eating raw meat (poultry) or through contact with the pathogen in the feces of other animals (pigeons, ducks). If a dog's resistance is adequate, infection doesn't necessarily lead to an outbreak of the disease.

Treatment: A good diet (see page 24) and antibiotics.

Tetanus

An infection caused by bacteria that enter the bloodstream through puncture wounds and then multiply and give off nerve toxins. Tetanus is quite rare in dogs, which is why there is no need for vaccinating them.

Course of the disease: At first, cramping of the muscles on the head because the toxins travel along the nerve paths to the spinal canal and to the brain. Vertical wrinkles appear on the forehead, the ears stand up erect, the corners of the mouth draw back, and the eyes narrow; heavy drooling because the dog is unable to swallow.

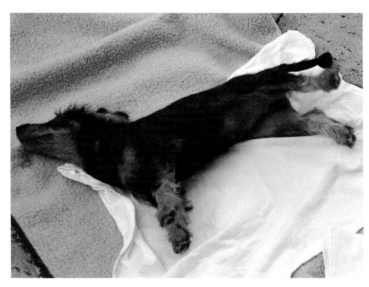

A dog suffering from tetanus. All the muscles are tensely cramped.

As the condition worsens, a high fever develops because of permanently cramped muscles, the tail gets stiff, the gait is stiff and awkward, and the dog lies down on its side.

Treatment: Tetanus anti-serum and antibiotics are inject-ed, and artificial feeding is nec-essary (because of the inability to swallow). Strong sedatives and narcotics given to relax the cramping and to induce a restful sleep (for 1 to 2 week) improve the chances of recovery. In spite of these measures, tetanus is sometimes fatal in dogs.

Toxoplasmosis

A disease caused by proto-zoans (see Glossary, page 118). Affects dogs *and* humans.

Course of the disease: The pathogen lives in the small intestine of cats, but humans and dogs can also catch the disease from cat feces infected with oocysts or—most com-monly—from eating uncooked meat, primarily pork, lamb, beef, and goat. In puppies and young dogs the disease causes severe infections accompanied by cough, purulent nasal dis-charge, vomiting and diarrhea, jaundice, pneumonia and heart and eye problems. In its chron-ic form, toxoplasmosis can, like distemper, lead to encephalitis.

Treatment: If the disease has not progressed too far, sulfa drugs and antibiotics given over 2 to 3 weeks are quite effective.

Diseases Caused by Parasites

There are two types of parasites:
• Ectoparasites (fleas, lice, mites, ticks) attack the outside of the body and lead to allergic reactions of the skin and strong itching.
• Endoparasites live in the intestines and in other internal organs and usually cause chron-ic disorders of these organs (see the appropriate sections in the various chapters). In the follow-ing pages, the typical symptoms and the method of transmission of the most common ectopara-sites are described, and, where appropriate, contagiousness to humans is mentioned.

Roundworms

Signs: Spaghetti-like worms (ascarids) 4 to 6 inches (10–15 cm) long found in the feces and in the vomit of the dog, or labo-ratory analysis of a stool sample showing worm eggs. The worms live in the small intestine.

Symptoms: Weight loss; diar-rhea with bloating, anemia, and, in puppies, interference with development. The larvae are carried in the blood stream to the liver and lungs where they can cause hepatitis, bron-chitis, and pneumonia.

Transmission: Puppies are generally already infected in the uterus through the mother's blood. Worms are found in their stool by the time they are

4 weeks old (see Deworming, page 21).

Contagiousness to humans: Through contact with worm eggs in dog feces.

Hookworms

Signs: Small, hook-shaped worms or worm eggs in the stool. The worms attach them-selves to the wall of the small intestine and suck blood.

Symptoms: Bloody diarrhea and pale mucous membranes.

Transmisstion: Dogs get hookworms through things they eat, or the larvae may burrow into the skin. Puppies absorb the larvae in their mother's milk from the 3rd week on. Migrating larvae occasionally cause lung problems (see Deworming, page 21).

Contagiousness to humans: People are very rarely infected because there is a different hook-worm that preys on humans.

Whipworms

Signs: Whip-shaped worms or worm eggs in the feces or in eggs deposited on fur by infect-ed dog when it licks itself.

Symptoms: Diarrhea, some-times bloody, and general weakness, especially in pup-pies; biting at flank.

Transmission: Through the food. Whipworms and hook-worms are often found in ken-nels and places where dealers keep their dogs (see Deworming, page 21).

Contagiousness to humans: People are rarely infected because there is a different whipworm that preys on humans.

Coccidia

Signs: Coccidia in laboratory analysis of stool samples.

Symptoms: Mucus-like diarrhea tinged with blood, especially in puppies and young dogs.

Transmission: Infected feces of other dogs or "carrier" mice that the dog eats.

Treatment: Sulfa drugs and antibiotics best given in two 5- to 6-day series with a period of 6 days in between.

Contagiousness to humans: None.

Tapeworms

Signs: Mobile body segments ³⁄₁₆ to ⅜ inch (5–10 mm) long and whitish, found in the dog's stool and the hairs around the anus.

Symptoms: Rough coat, intermittent diarrhea, weight loss in spite of good appetite, itchy anus.

Transmission: Primarily through ingestion of raw meat and internal organs of beef, goat, sheep, and deer but also through eating mice, rats, and fleas. These intermediary hosts are in turn infected by dog and cat feces and fox droppings. The most common tapeworm of dogs uses fleas as intermediary host. That is why deworming is important if a dog is infested with fleas. The so-called fox

tapeworm is extremely rare in dogs. See Deworming, page 21.

Contagiousness to humans: Rare with normal hygiene. It is possible for humans to be "mistakenly" adopted as intermediary host by dog, cat, or fox tapeworms after contact with worm eggs.

Lungworms

Signs: Laboratory analysis reveals larvae in the feces.

Symptoms: Bronchitis and pneumonia (see page 55).

Transmission: Through larvae in the feces of other dogs.

Treatment: Injection of appropriate drugs effective against the parasite.

Contagiousness to humans: None.

Imported Diseases

Not only people but dogs as well can return from travels to tropical and subtropical regions with tropical diseases. But these diseases are more common in dogs imported from these parts of the world. The pathogens are minute blood parasites transmitted by flies, mosquitoes, or ticks.

Leishmaniasis

Pathogen: A protozoan that lives in the blood of dogs. It is transmitted by sand flies or enters the body through open wounds.

Distribution: Mediterranean, northern Africa, central Europe.

Symptoms: Hair loss, excessive dandruff, eczema all over the body, swollen lymph nodes, bouts of fever, general weakness, weight loss, bloated belly. Incubation period (see Glossary, page 117) is 3 to 6 months.

Treatment: Very costly and effective only in the early stages. The sickness often flares up again after apparent cure.

Contagiousness to humans: There is a danger of transmission via minor scratches and wounds! Consider having the dog put to sleep if the disease has reached an advanced stage.

Babesiasis (Piroplasmosis)

Pathogen: A tiny protozoan that destroys red blood cells and causes anemia; transmitted by ticks.

Distribution: Tropical and subtropical countries; central Europe.

Symptoms: Ten to 20 days after exposure, tiredness, weakness, bouts of high fever, pale mucous membranes, dark urine, jaundice.

Treatment: Drugs that combat this pathogen are likely to lead to recovery.

Contagiousness to humans: None.

Canine Rickettsiosis (Ehrlichsiosis)

Pathogen: A bacteria-like blood parasite that destroys white blood cells and weakens the immune system. Transmitted by ticks.

Distribution: Tropical and subtropical countries, central Europe.

Symptoms: Rickettsiosis often coincides with babesiasis and produces similar symptoms but in a more virulent form.

Treatment: Drugs used against babesiasis or antibiotics are likely to lead to recovery.

Contagiousness to humans: None.

Heartworms
Pathogen: A worm 1 millimeter in diameter and up to 10 inches (25 cm) long that lives in the right atrium of the heart and in the arteries of the lungs. It causes serious heart and lung problems. The larvae are transmitted by mosquitoes.

Distribution: Southern North America, Central America, Mediterranean.

Symptoms: Decline of energy, coughing, heart and circulatory problems accompanied by congestion of the lungs; faster than normal breathing and pulse rate.

Treatment: The veterinarian injects a drug containing arsenic against the adult worms. Dogs are given heartworm pills once a month as a preventive measure.

Contagiousness to humans: Rare, unless an infected mosquito bites a human.

Disorders Associated with Certain Breeds

Breeders' ambition and the pride of owners have in the course of time produced more and more outlandish dog breeds—anything from miniature dogs with pushed-in noses or short legs to huge and heavy ones. The risk of hereditary diseases that goes along with this kind of breeding is well known. We can only hope that the desire to produce not just beautiful but also healthy dogs will continue to grow stronger. In the following paragraphs the breeds that commonly develop diseases brought on by mating animals from lines that are too closely related are listed along with their typical diseases.

Toy Breeds
Toy versions of the Yorkshire terrier, Shih Tzu, Chihuahua, miniature pinscher, poodle, and schnauzer commonly suffer from
• deformities of the knee and hip joints (see pages 88 to 93);
• collapsed windpipe because of cartilage malformations (see page 54);
• incomplete change from puppy to permanent teeth, tendency to develop periodontosis (see page 40);
• problems during delivery because of narrow pelvis.

Short-nosed Breeds
Pugs, Pekingese, Boston terriers, and French bulldogs are susceptible to
• breathing difficulties and rhinitis (see page 52) because of shortened nose;
• inflammation and infections in the throat and larynx (see page 53). Danger of choking to death if a dog gets highly excited or if it is very hot because of too narrow an oral opening, and too large a soft palate and tongue;
• problems during delivery because the puppies' heads are too large.

An Extreme of Breeders' Fancy
The Chinese fighting dog Shar Pei (see drawing, page 78) has through selective breeding acquired excessively large and numerous skin folds. This breed suffers from
• eye problems because the eye slit is too narrow (see page 75);
• weeping eczema in the skin folds (see page 80).

Big Dogs
The problems big dogs, such as the German shepherd, Saint Bernard, basset hound, Bernese mountain dog, mastiff, Rottweiler, and Great Dane, suffer from are:
• deformities of the hip and elbow joints (see pages 88 and 91);
• herniated discs (see page 94);
• heart disease (see page 59);
• conjunctivitis in dogs with "watery eyes" because the eye slit is too wide (see page 75).

Behavioral Problems

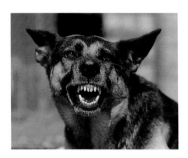

A dog may bite a member of the family, love to get into dog fights, disappear for days at a time, or drive the neighbors to distraction with its incessant barking—in short, it behaves in ways people find unacceptable. We speak in these cases of behavioral problems or abnormal behavior.

These problems arise from over-breeding, unnatural conditions during the puppy's imprinting phase, and incorrect training and handling of the dog—generally because the owners don't know enough about the nature of dogs and therefore don't treat them properly.

How to Avoid Behavioral Problems

Dogs are pack animals by nature and as such are used to a strict rank hierarchy. A domestic dog wants to have its place in the "pack" of the family clearly defined. It needs an authority to which it can submit. This doesn't mean that the dog should be beaten into a sumissive creature—quite the contrary. Not only bullies but overly timid dogs, too, which sometimes bite out of fear, are examples of abnormal behavior.

Proper dog training is approached with love but also with firmness. Praise and discipline are used to reinforce good behavior and to link, in the dog's mind, improper behavior with an unpleasant experience, which may be

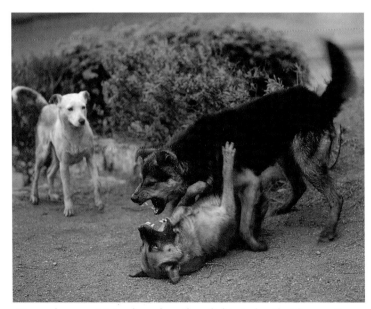

Dogs observe strict rules when they fight. A dog that lies on its back signals by this gesture that it is giving up.

nothing more than a loud verbal reproof. Being beaten is not a form of physical punishment a dog understands; instead, shake the animal briefly by the scruff of the neck, the way the mother does when teaching the puppy.

It is in the nature of dogs to try constantly to improve their rank within their social group. If a human being fails to assert over and over again the claim to the top slot, the dog will usurp the leadership role and soon rule over and tyrannize the entire family. We speak in this case of "dominance aggression." It means that the dog acts as if it were the boss and defends certain areas (the sofa or the kitchen), growling or even biting if anyone intrudes into these territories.

Some simple training exercises help to prevent things coming to such a pass. If you notice that the dog obeys only reluctantly, that it transgresses limits it has been taught—getting up on a forbidden couch, for example—you should practice exercises in which the dog has to submit itself. Go through the "Sit," "Come," and "Stay" exercises the dog learned as a puppy and insist on perfect obedience to the commands. Praise the dog when it performs properly and discipline it if it resists. If the dog ignores commands as soon as it is beyond your reach, throw something with which you can hit it but not hurt it (such as a tennis ball) to show it that you are still in command.

Dealing with Behavioral Problems

If you find that your dog is displaying serious behavioral problems, such as aggression toward other dogs as well as against people, fits of destructiveness, breaking loose and roaming, you should consult your veterinarian. Sometimes castration or drugs can help. If the problem is inadequate training, the veterinarian will recommend a dog obedience school. In big cities there are also animal psychiatrists.

Consistent reeducation may be necessary to deal with behavioral problems. You should in this case consult a professional dog trainer. Anyone who has allowed things to get to the point where a dog disregards its master's authority is usually not strong-willed enough to exercise the firmness necessary to correct the mistakes. In any case, both the dog and its owner will have to do some major relearning. In exceptionally problematic cases, professional dog trainers sometimes successfully use a collar that can emit electric impulses. However, nobody should use this device without professional advice.

Castration—the Solution to Many Problems

American experiments have shown that castration (see Glossary, page 115) resolves certain behavior problems in male dogs. Aggression between males, for example, was reduced in about 60% of the subjects, and roaming decreased in about 90%. Castration is also likely to reduce hypersexuality and urine marking.

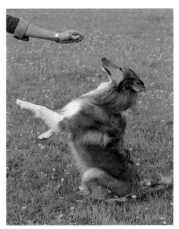

Regular repetition of lessons learned is a good method of training.

Estrus and Birth

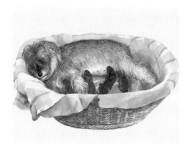

*O*ur family has just experienced a significant increase in numbers: Nelly has given birth to four puppies, little black bundles of life that fit into the hollow of your hand. We tiptoe up to the birthing box to watch Nelly lick her babies now that their little bellies are full and they have dropped off to sleep. Nelly leaves the basket only when she has to relieve herself. She returns instantly, and it looks as though she were counting her young. We can tell that she is a good mother, and we, too, want to do our best by them and find good homes for them.

Estrus

A female dog reaches sexual maturity at 6 to 9 months. After that she goes into heat twice a year. It is during this season of heat—and only then—that female dogs mate. The heat cycle lasts 2 to 3 weeks and has two distinct phases.

During the first phase, or proestrus, which lasts about 9–12 days, the dog is restless, and there is a bloody discharge from the vagina. The male dogs in the neighborhood already detect the scent and approach the bitch with great interest. She, however, rejects all their overtures because she is not yet ready.

• This situation changes during the second phase of estrus, the standing heat. The vaginal bleeding diminishes and the female is more tolerant of her admirers. She lets herself be sniffed, stands still, and moves her tail aside when a male meets her fancy. This is a clear signal that she is ready to mate. If you don't want puppies, this is the time when you have to keep a sharp eye out.

The Mating

Many people are amazed, when they see dogs mating, how long the pair stays locked together during sexual intercourse. The union can last as much as 15 to 30 minutes. It is very important not to try to separate them by force during this phase. This would not only be

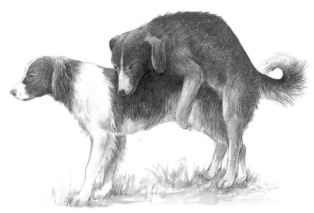

When copulating, dogs remain locked together for 15 to 30 minutes. Never try to separate them by force!

very painful but also cause physical injury and bleeding.

A bitch is receptive for a period of a few days. If she mates with several males during this time the offspring of the same litter quite commonly have different fathers.

Pregnancy

During the 3rd or 4th week a veterinarian can tell by feeling the dog's belly if she is pregnant. From the 6th week on, X-rays show how many puppies may be expected. Some animal clinics now even offer ultrasound tests that do not rely upon ionizing radiation.

Diet during pregnancy: The gestation period of dogs is 60 to 65 days. During this time the dog gets lazier, hungrier, and fatter by the day. To keep her and the future puppies in good health, it is important to feed her especially well during this time. In the last few weeks of pregnancy, she will need twice or three times the ration she ordinarily gets, and her food has to be rich in minerals, trace elements, and vitamins (see pages 14 and 15). Toward the end of gestation and during the nursing period the supplements have to contain plenty of calcium. Your veterinarian or any pet store will sell you appropriate vitamin and mineral supplements.

Toward the end of pregnancy the bitch wants to prepare a nest, and you should therefore have the birthing box ready in good time.

False Pregnancy

As also discussed on page 72, the first signs of a false pregnancy show up about two months after estrus. The bitch behaves as if she were raising puppies. In wild animals that live in packs, such as wolves, false pregnancy serve a useful function: If a mother is unable to take care of her puppies for whatever reason, there is always a surrogate mother ready to take her place and suckle them. In the conditions under which our modern domestic dogs live, false pregnancy has an adverse effect on the dog's health (see pages 72 and 73). Her breasts fill with milk and there is no use for it. This often leads to mastitis, which leaves behind small lumps in the mammary glands. If a bitch undergoes false pregnancy after every heat cycle, spaying (see Glossary, page 119) should be considered as a cancer preventive measure.

Getting Ready for the Birth

A bitch needs a quiet spot where she can deliver and raise her young. Put the birthing box in this place during the dog's pregnancy so that she can get used to it.

You can construct a birthing box out of some boards. For small dogs, a basket works fine. The rule of thumb is that the

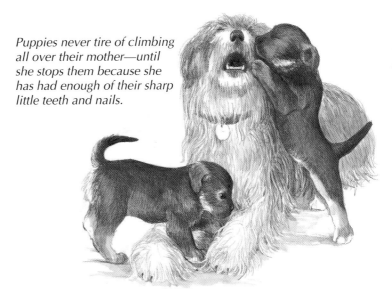

Puppies never tire of climbing all over their mother—until she stops them because she has had enough of their sharp little teeth and nails.

height of the box should be about a third of the dog's shoulder height and that the area should be about three times the area the dog takes up when lying down. Line the box with a cloth or blanket, but make sure there are no holes or fringes in which the puppies might get caught.

A heat lamp with an infra-red 150-watt bulb should be installed above the box to keep the temperature 85–90°F in one corner of the box for the first 7 days. Raise the bulb about 20 to 32 inches (50–80 cm) above the bottom of the box and mount it in such a way that the dog can't knock it down. The lamp is important because puppies can't maintain their body heat by themselves during the first weeks of life and therefore need a constant source of warmth, especially if the mother leaves the box frequently.

The Birth

Healthy bitches usually give birth without problems and without human assistance. However, there are some tiny breeds, such as the Yorkshire terrier and the Pekingese, which are often unable to deliver naturally. If your dog belongs to this risk group, consult your veterinarian. He or she might suggest a caesarean section.

In a normal birth the puppies appear one at a time about ½ to 1 hour apart. The mother eats the fetal membrane and the placenta and bites off the umbilical cord (see pictures 1 to 4). There is a good reason for this: The placenta contains hormones that speed up the birthing process and the secretion of milk. And by licking the puppies, the mother also stimulates the circulation of the puppies, which are still blind but immediately and instinctively head for the nipples.

When assistance is needed: Even if the delivery is going normally you should still watch the bitch. Help is called for if the mother neglects to remove the transparent fetal membrane; the puppy might suffocate. Open the membrane, tie off the umbilical cord with dental floss, and cut off with scissors, leaving about 1 inch (2–3 cm) beyond the floss ligature. Then place the puppy in front of the mother so she will lick it.

You should also be concerned if more than an hour passes before the next puppy appears. You probably know how many puppies to expect from the veterinarian's examination of the dog. Call the veterinarian if labor comes to a standstill. Perhaps one of the puppies has too large a head or it may be in breech position.

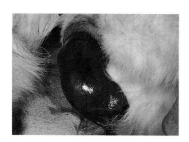

1. The emerging puppy is still inside the fetal membrane.

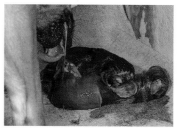

2. The mother bites the membrane open and eats it.

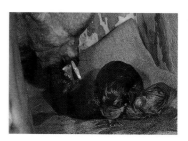

3. The mother bites the umbilical cord off and licks the puppy clean.

Raising the Puppies

The mother takes care of her puppies all by herself for the first 4 weeks. All you have to do during this time is check to make sure that all of them are getting enough milk and that the stronger don't push the weaker ones off the nipples. The milk secreted during the first few days, the colostrum, is especially important for building up the puppies' immune resistance.

From the 5th week on you have to supplement the mother's milk with solid food, and you have to start cleaning the birthing box because once the puppies start eating food the mother stops eating their feces. In the 6th week the puppies should get dewormed. After a second deworming the puppies get their first immunizations during the 8th week (see page 20). Then, when they are 8 or 9 weeks old, the puppies can be given to their new owners.

If You Don't Want Puppies

Many people think that a female dog should be allowed, for the sake of her health, to have puppies once. This is a misconception. There are many reasons why dog owners choose not to breed their dogs. One very good reason is that shelters everywhere are filled with homeless dogs. If you want your bitch not to have puppies you have several methods to choose from:

• If the bitch is already pregnant, you can take her to the veterinarian, who can give her three hormone injections 2 days apart. This is, however, an emergency solution and shouldn't be routinely resorted to after every heat cycle. The danger of pyometra, ovarian cysts, and tumors is too great.
• Prevention is always preferable. There are hormone injections that, if given regularly every 4 to 5 months, prevent the bitch from going into heat. This is, of course, not an ideal solution either because hormone injections always increase the risk of pyometra, ovarian tumors, and breast cancer.
• Spaying is the only sensible route to go if one wants to permanently prevent estrus and pregnancy and is concerned about the dog's health not just now but until old age. In this operation the ovaries and most of the uterus are removed. This, of course, also eliminates the risk of diseases affecting these

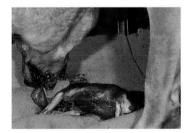

4. The mother's licking tongue also stimulates the puppy's circulation.

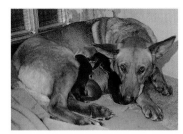

5. Guided by instinct, the puppies have located the milk-filled nipples.

organs. The earlier a dog is spayed—about 4 to 6 months of age is ideal—the smaller the chance that the dog will develop breast cancer.

About spaying: It is not true that dogs become lazy after being spayed. Because of the change in hormone production they are hungry and consequently become fatter and slower-moving. But if you reduce the food ration by a third, this problem doesn't arise. The dog won't gain weight or get lazy.

Aftereffects of spaying: The texture of the coat may change. Longhaired, reddish fur, in particular, tends to get fluffier. Large dogs may in old age develop a problem controlling urination. This form of incontinence responds to hormone treatments.

Old Dogs

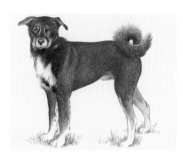

*Y*our dog is slowly turning gray: White hairs appear first along the lips and on the chin, then on the cheeks and nose and around the eyes; and finally the forehead and the entire head turn gray. Your dog has gotten old. Hearing and eyesight begin to fail, but luckily the nose, through which the dog "experiences" the world, still works fine in old age. Running is more of an effort than it used to be, but sometimes your old dog still frolics almost like a puppy. There may be occasional lapses in house training—a natural and forgivable weakness in old age.

When Does a Dog Get Old?

One year in the life of a dog is the equivalent of several human years. The first year is comparable to about 15 years for humans, the second to only about 8, and from the 3rd year on, each year should be multiplied by 4 (see table on page 111).

As a general rule one can say that large dogs live considerably less than medium-sized and small ones. Boxers, Great Danes, and Saint Bernards, for example, generally live to about 10 to 12, whereas poodles, dachshunds, and fox terriers may easily reach an age of 16 to 18 years. Strains bred to be exceptionally small, such as the toy versions of the Yorkshire terrier, poodle, Pomeranian, and schnauzer, usually don't get to be as old as their medium-sized relatives.

Diet

The metabolism of an old dog is no longer able to make as efficient use of food as when it was younger. And the digestion no longer functions as well because internal organs, such as the intestines, liver, and pancreas, begin to show signs of wearing out.

Amount of food: Since old dogs are no longer as active as they used to be, the food ration should be reduced. A good rule of thumb is: no more than 7 ounces (200 g) per 20 pounds (10 kg) of body weight per day.

Menu composition: You should give an old dog the following foods:

Mostly easily digestible carbohydrates, such as brown rice, dog food meal, potatoes, or noodles—foods that are also rich in minerals and vitamins (about ⅔ of the ration).

Meat should not make up more than ⅓ of the ration and should consist of high-quality, easily digestible proteins, such as lean meat, poultry, or fish.

Milk products, such as low-fat or fat-free cottage cheese, are also a good source of protein.

Obesity is as big a problem for old dogs as for people. That's why you should sometimes give your dog specially prepared commercial diets formulated for the aging canine.

Important: Since old dogs tend to develop kidney problems, you should add a little salt or garlic/onion powder to the food and make it tasty with some meat broth since the high proportion of carbohydrates otherwise makes the food taste bland and uninteresting. Salt has to be reduced only if a dog has heart problems.

Fluid requirements: Make sure your dog is drinking enough. An old dog should drink about 1 pint (½ l) of water

Comparison of Dog Years and Human Years

Age of a Dog	Age of a Person
1 year	15 years
2 years	23 years
3 years	27 years
4 years	31 years
5 years	35 years
and so on	and so on

per 20 pounds (10 kg) of body weight. About 75% of this is absorbed in the wet food, but the rest (about 4 ounces or 125 ml) the dog has to ingest in the form of water. If you feed your dog primarily on dry food, it should drink about 1 cup (¼ l) per 20 pounds (10 kg) of body weight.

Diseases of Old Age

The natural wear and tear accumulating in the course of a dog's life plus the effects on the body of diseases and injuries the dog has sustained can give rise to a number of infirmities in old age. Old age itself, however, is not a disease! It is not uncommon for dog owners to come to the veterinarian to have their old pet put to sleep just because it suffers from some health problem that would have responded to treatment or could even have been cured altogether. As the animal's owner you are responsible for your dog's life. That is why you should look after your dog with special care as it gets old. Watch for symptoms that signal the onset of a health problem and don't wait to take the dog to the veterinarian until it's too late for sensible treatment.

Problems Moving

The joints are the weak spots in an aging dog. The effects of wear and tear cause chronic arthritis (see page 92), and often there are problems with herniated disks as well (see page 94). The dog will move stiffly especially after lying down for some time. It first has to "warm up."

You can help by covering the dog when it sleeps and by making sure the sleeping place is not too hard and cold. Keep the dog from overstraining the problematic joints. It's better to take 3 or 4 short walks a day than one hour-long hike. Also, prevent your dog from getting carried away when you throw a ball or stick for it, take it along bicycling, or let it play with other dogs.

Problems of the Circulatory System

Older dogs quite commonly develop chronic heart problems (see page 59). Such dogs should get medication to strengthen the heart and should be kept from overexerting and getting too excited. Also try to avoid exposure to humid heat.

You can help by keeping the dog's exercise within bounds and calming it when it gets excited. Remember, for example, that the exuberance with which it greets you might be too much, and that the dog might faint from excitement. Try, therefore, to calm the dog rather than spur it on. Also remember that a dog with heart problems should get very little salt in its food.

Chronic Disorders of the Internal Organs

Chronic kidney or liver problems are not uncommon in old dogs that earlier suffered infections or poisonings. Excessive thirst, occasional vomiting, and soft stool can be early signs of these problems.

You can help by making sure the dog does not overexert or get too excited. Keep it on a strict diet (see page 24).

If they are given proper care and are checked regularly by the veterinarian, dogs with chronic problems of this kind can still live quite happily for several years.

Skin Problems

With advancing age, skin disorders also tend to be on the increase. They take the form of hair loss, increased flakiness, more warts, and, other skin tumors, which are, however, generally benign.

You can help by having the veterinarian remove in good time warts and lumps growing from sebaceous glands. If the dog scratches these places too much, they can get inflamed and spread. Old boxers especially should have skin tumors checked as promptly as possible because this breed tends to develop malignant tumors (see page 24).

Hormonal Problems

Hair loss occurring in a symmetrical pattern on the body and the thighs generally indicates some hormonal imbalance. Inadequate output of thyroid hormones (see page 85) or hyperfunction of the adrenal cortex (see page 86) often occur only as a dog gets old. Excessive thirst—the dog drinks more than 1 pint (1 l) of water per 20 pounds (10 kg) of body weight a day—is often the first indication of diabetes (see page 87).

Special Health Problems of Old Female Dogs

If a female dog is not spayed, her estrus cycles will, as she gets older, often become irregular because of hormonal problems. Prolonged bleeding and inflammation or infection of the uterus (see page 72) may be the result.

You can help by watching your dog closely. If you notice a vaginal discharge, increased thirst, and a general decline in health 6 to 8 weeks after estrus, take the dog to the veterinarian without delay. Also get in the habit of feeling the dog's breasts when you pet her. If you feel any hard places, consult the veterinarian promptly. Caused by repeated false pregnancies (see page 72), lumps often form in the breasts of older bitches and should be operated on promptly.

Special Health Problems of Old Male Dogs

Enlarged prostates are common primarily in hypersexual males (see page 67). This condition leads to difficulties passing stool and sometimes to bloody urine.

You can help by having your dog neutered.

Caring for an Old Dog

Your dog needs some special preventive health care in old age. Regular grooming of the

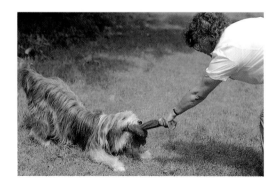

Play keeps even an old dog "young" and helps it get needed exercise.

coat and cleaning of the ears, teeth, paws, and anal and genital region become increasingly important as the dog grows older.

Regular Care

With advancing years dogs develop more tartar on their teeth (see page 40), which contributes to periodontitis as well as to loosening and infection of the teeth. This can be prevented through regular dental care. Give your dog enough bones (the best are the ball part of ball-and-socket joints of veal or beef; do not give him poultry or hollow bones) and dog biscuits for natural cleaning of the teeth, and clean its teeth if necessary. You can buy special tooth paste and tooth brushes from your veterinarian or at pet stores.

When grooming the coat, check the dog's body all over for warts and lumps. Effective treatment by the veterinarian depends on early recognition.

When cleaning the various bodily orifices, watch for dirt from secretions and for lumps or tumors that might be forming. Here, too, close observation helps to spot disease at an early stage.

Preventive Health Checks

Regular physical examinations are a good idea for dogs as well as for people. Chronic diseases of the various organs, hormonal malfunctionings, and developing tumors are thus discovered and can be treated early. When you take your dog for its annual immunization (see Vaccination Schedule, page 20), the veterinarian can check the dog all over.

Dogs over 8 years old should be checked twice a year. The examination should include a urine test, a blood analysis, and a careful check of the heart.

• A urine sample (which the owner should bring along) will show if the dog has diabetes, kidney problems, or liver disease.

• Various blood analyses (see Glossary, page 115) indicate chronic kidney, liver, and hormonal problems.

• Regular checking of the heart is important for dogs and helps improve their longevity. Heart disease can often be detected by abnormal sounds of the heart long before it manifests itself in other symptoms. By checking the dog regularly and watching the symptoms which gradually lead to circulatory problems, the veterinarian can determine in consultation with you when is the right time to initiate measures to assist the heart.

Thanks to the consistent efforts of dog owners in taking proper care of their pets, initiating preventive measures such as immunization and deworming, observing closely and spotting symptoms promptly, and taking their animals in for detailed physical check-ups dogs now live an average of 2 to 3 years longer than they used to.

Important: Keep in mind that old age is not a disease and that many diseases of old age can be treated or managed quite successfully.

The Last Trip to the Veterinarian

When the time has finally come when modern medicine can no longer prolong your dog's life, you should release the animal from its suffering and have it put to sleep (euthanasia).

The veterinarian injects a fatal dose of an anesthetic agent, usually directly into a vein, so that the dog feels no pain and goes to sleep peacefully. After the many years it has lived with you in loyalty and friendship, you owe it to your dog to let it die painlessly. You also owe it your company on this last journey to the veterinarian so that the dog may rest its head in your hand as it is given this final injection. Of course this decision is up to the owner, who may find the experience too distressing.

Glossary

In the course of discussing his or her pet's health or illness with the veterinarian, a dog owner often hears technical terms whose meaning is not always obvious. But there is no reason why you should not be able to understand the vocabulary veterinarians use. In the following pages some of the most important terms are explained.

Aerosol
Medication in the form of a spray (the solid or liquid particles of the drug are suspended in a gas) used for inhalation therapy (qv).

Allergens
Substances that induce allergy.

Analgesics
Drugs that relieve pain.

Anconeal process
An extension of the ulna in the elbow joint that sometimes is not properly attached or tears off and causes arthritis.

Angiography
Radiographic visualization of blood vessels by means of X-rays (qv) or fluoroscopy (qv) after injection of a contrast medium that appears opaque on film or on the fluoroscope.

Antacids
Medications to relieve overacidity of the stomach.

Antibiotics
Medications that inhibit the reproduction of bacteria or protozoans (qv).

Antibodies
Specific proteins formed by the immune system of the body to fight specific pathogens.

Antidote
A substance that counteracts the effects of poison.

Antihistamines
Medications given to suppress allergic reactions.

Anti-inflammatories
Medications that counteract inflammation.

Antimycotics (Antifungals)
Medications that inhibit the growth of fungi.

Asepsis
Sterility; absence of germs on medical instruments or surfaces to be surgically invaded. Objects can be made aseptic by heating them to 290°F (160°C) and keeping them at that temperature in a dry sterilizer for at least 2 hours. Patient's surfaces are prepared for aseptic surgery by thorough cleansing and application of antiseptics.

Atrioventricular Valves
The valves between the atrium and the ventriculum in both sides of the heart that regulate the blood flow.

Aujeszky's disease
Pseudorabies. Caused by a virus found mostly in pigs. Dogs contract the disease most commonly by eating undercooked pork. Pseudorabies is fatal for dogs, but it is not transmissible to humans. The symptoms resemble those of rabies (see page 99).

Bacterial examination
The checking of smears and staining for the presence of bacteria.

Biopsy
Removal of a bit of tissue with a scalpel, through a hollow needle, or with tiny forceps (see Endoscopy). The tissue is then processed and stained in the laboratory and examined under the microscope.

Blood analysis (Chemistry panel)
Establishment of the amounts of certain substances in the blood,

such as blood sugar, urea, cholesterol, electrolytes, and enzymes.

Blood count (Complete)
Analysis of how many red and the distribution of what kinds of white blood corpuscles there are in a given volume of blood; the amount of hemoglobin and the nature of plasma in the sample.

Breed
A group of dogs with a common ancestry and with certain typical traits (breed standards) that are arbitrarily defined by the particular breed associations. External appearance is of primary importance, and in the pursuit of perfect appearance, degeneration as well as congenital defects are often considered acceptable risks.

Broad-spectrum antibiotics
Antibiotics that are effective against many kinds of germs.

Bronchodilators
Drugs that dilate the airways.

Canine teeth
The big corner teeth in both the upper and the lower jaw that serve to get hold of the prey. In small breeds, the deciduous (baby) canines are often retained as the adult teeth

erupt. If the baby teeth can't be loosened, they should be pulled under anesthesia by the time the puppy is 9 months old at the latest.

Castration
Surgical removal of a male dog's testicles to reduce aggressiveness or hypersexuality or because of prostate troubles or tumors on the testes.

Chemotherapeutic (Cytostatic) drugs
Medications that retard cellular multiplication and are used to fight cancer.

Cirrhosis of the liver
Also called fibrosis of the liver. Chronic liver disease caused by toxins or other harmful substances leads to degeneration and death of liver cells. In a kind of scarring process the dead cells are replaced by fibrous tissue. As a result the liver becomes hard and shriveled.

Clostridial infection
Infection of a wound with bacteria that produce gas and/or toxins (Clostridia). Examples are tetanus, gas gangrene, and botulism.

Computer tomography
A diagnostic technique in

which X-ray pictures taken at different focal lengths are electronically processed and analyzed in such a way that they yield cross section images of the body.

Cortisone
A drug similar in nature and effect to the hormone cortisol produced by the adrenal cortex. It has been much overprescribed because of its effectiveness in reducing inflammation and itching, improving appetite, relieving pain, and as a stimulant. Cortisone is irreplaceable, however, for relieving chronic skin and joint problems.

Decongestants
Drugs that loosen and dissolve the mucus produced in the airways by bronchial inflammation. The mucus can then be coughed up more easily.

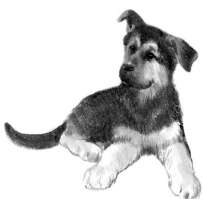

Dehydration
Drying out of the body tissue because of fluid loss. If the skin of a dog in this condition is pulled up, the skin fold "stands up" tent-like for a while.

Desensitization
The skin is rendered less sensitive to allergies through drugs especially formulated for this purpose and usually given in a series of injections.

Disorders of the central nervous system
Motor and sensory disturbances originating in the brain or the spinal cord. Staggering, stiff or weaving gait, convulsions, epileptic fits.

Dispensing privileges
Permission veterinarians have not only to prescribe medicines but also to prepare and sell them. Unlike physicians for humans, veterinarians may legally run a pharmacy.

Diuretics
Drugs that increase the flow of urine from the kidneys.

Docking tails and cropping ears
These cosmetic procedures are performed in certain breeds to achieve, for example, the erect ears of boxers, Great Danes, and Dobermans and the stub tails of boxers and schnauzers. Cropping of ears was declared illegal in several European countries in 1990. The tail is best docked in puppies under 4 days of age.

Draining
Allowing the secretion from a wound to flow off through an opening lined with a gauze strip or though a small rubber tube.

Dyspnea
Labored respiration experienced either when breathing in (respiratory dyspnea) or out (exhalatory dyspnea).

Edema
Accumulation of fluid in the tissue of the lungs and skin.

Electrocardiogram
Abbreviation: ECG. A graph tracing the electrical impulses involved in the heart's activity.

Electrolytes
Salts and minerals, such as sodium, potassium, calcium, chloride, phosphorus, and magnesium that have to be present in certain concentrations in the body fluids.

Embryonic development
Growth of the embryo in the uterus from the first cell division after fertilization of the egg to the maturing of a viable organism shortly before birth.

Endoscopy
A method of physical examination in which an optical instrument is introduced into hollow organs (such as the stomach, intestine, or bladder), which thus become accessible to visual examination. Biopsies (qv) can be taken by the same method.

Extraction
Pulling out, as of a tooth.

Fatty liver disease
Buildup of fatty tissue in the liver. Initially the fat provides some protection against poisons, which it absorbs, thereby protecting liver cells. But if the liver is constantly overloaded with fat, the process perpetuates itself and leads to fatty degeneration of the liver.

Fluoroscopy
Longer exposure of body regions to electronically magnified X-rays. Movements within the body become visible on a screen and can be recorded on video.

Folliculitis
Superficial, purulent inflammation of the hair pores.

Health insurance
In recent years insurance companies have started offering health insurance policies for

dogs and cats. A portion of the costs for preventive measures, such as vaccinations and deworming are also reimbursed. Animals can be insured from age 4 months on but may be no older than 5 years when the policy is issued.

Heterosis effect
Increased vitality as a result of crossbreeding. If dogs of different breeds or of mixed breeds are crossbred, the offspring show increased disease resistance and fertility.

Icterus
Jaundice. Yellow discoloration of the mucous membranes and the skin because of an increase in the blood of bile pigments. Generally the result of liver damage.

Immune fluorescence
Investigative method in which fluorescent antibodies in sections of the skin are examined under the microscope. These antibodies indicate autoimmune disorders.

Inbreeding
The mating of closely related animals. This happens commonly in nature and may have no effect in the first generation of offspring. But if lines that are too closely related are consistently mated, this can result in so-called genetic defects. By

crossing in other breeds and backcrossing these mixed-breed dogs with the original breed, such defects can be avoided.

Incarcerated hernia
Painful binding of protruded organ in a hernia and growing together of tissue that tends to become inflamed.

Incubation period
The period between exposure to and outbreak of a disease.

Inhalation therapy
Exposure to vapors (camomile, for example) or aerosols (qv) that are inhaled.

Injection
The giving of shots of medication into the veins (intravenous), into a muscle (intramuscular), under the skin (subcutaneous), into the mouth (oral), or into the rectum (rectal).

Insecticides
Also pesticides. Poisons used to combat parasites (insects, ticks, and mites).

Intravenous (fluid) therapy
Treatment with fluids that contain minerals (electrolytes) and glucose among other substances. The fluids are injected into the veins.

Internal bone fixation
Surgical method of setting fractures.

Intestinal flora
Colonies of bacteria in the intestines necessary for proper digestion.

Killed vaccine
Vaccine containing dead pathogens.

Lethal factor
A gene that may cause stillbirths or high mortality rate in puppies. The term semi-lethal factor is used if an animal dies of a congenital disease before reaching sexual maturity or before the age of 6 months. Often breeders knowingly accept the risk posed by a lethal factor in order to achieve a particular desired trait, such as white spots in tiger dachshunds.

Liability insurance
The owner is liable if an animal he or she owns kills or injures a person or damages property. Every dog owner should have insurance against such eventualities. A liability policy for dog ownership provides coverage if a dog, for example, causes an accident crossing the road, bites another dog, or pulls a person off a bicycle. The coverage does not apply to dogs that are deliberately trained to attack people.

Lithotripsy
A non-surgical method of pulverization of bladder stones by

means of shock waves produced by a lithotriptor machine.

Live vaccine
A vaccine containing living but attenuated, or weakened, pathogens.

Metastasis
Secondary cancers sent out by malignant tumors to other parts of the body (especially the lungs, spleen, liver, kidneys, and bone marrow); disseminated spread of a disease process.

Mixed breed
A dog that is not purebred. The heterosis effect (qv) is responsible for the fact that these dogs are often healthier and more resistant to disease than purebred dogs.

Molars
Big teeth in back of jaws used to chew and break up big pieces of food.

Mucopurulent
Referring to a discharge containing mucus and pus.

Necrosis
Atrophy or death of tissue, usually resulting from insufficient blood supply.

Neutering
Castration (see term) or spaying (see term).

Nocardiosis
Infestation of the lungs or deeper skin layers with a kind of bacteria *(Nocardia)* that grow like fungi (pseudomycelium). The infestation leads to pneumonia and abscesses in the skin that keep erupting and that have to be excised by removing large areas of skin.

The condition also has to be treated for weeks with antibiotics. Inside the body the pathogen causes severe, bloody, and putrescent infections in the thoracic and abdominal cavities.

Plasma expander
An artificial blood plasma introduced intravenously in cases of blood loss to maintain blood pressure; the plasma expander breaks down slowly.

Protozoans
Microscopic, usually unicellular organisms that can cause infections.

Purulent
Referring to pus; a pus-producing inflammatory process; usually an infection.

Pylorus
The muscles controlling the opening and closing mechanism between the stomach and the duodenum.

Quarantine
Isolation of animals that are sick or suspected of carrying a contagious disease; used to prevent epidemics.

Resistance (Immunity)
The ability of the body to fight off infections.

Resorption
Assimilation. Body tissues have the capacity to absorb fluids, air, and drugs and to distribute them throughout the body.

Scooting
A dog "scoots" by assuming a sitting position, stretching the hindlegs up, and dragging itself along the ground with the forelegs. Dogs do this if the anal region is itchy or sticky, if the anal glands are plugged, and occasionally if they have worms.

Secondary infection
An infection caused by bacteria or fungi in an organism weakened by an initial infection that is usually viral.

Secretion
The release of fluids from certain organs, such as the pancreas and the sebaceous and anal glands.

Serologic tests
The checking for presence in the blood of antibodies to

specific diseases. If the serum tests positive, the dog has previously encountered and produced antibodies to the pathogen in question.

Shrunken kidney
A kidney that has shrunk as a result of numerous infections. The original tissue of the organ is replaced by fibrous scar tissue.

Skin scraping
Scraping off of skin layers down to the dermis in order to examine these samples under the microscope for signs of parasites and fungi.

Spasmolytic drugs
Medication that relieves spasms.

Spaying
Surgical removal of a female dog's ovaries and uterus to prevent estrus, pregnancy, and false pregnancy. It is also used as a preventive procedure to reduce the chance of breast and uterine cancer and inflammation of the uterus.

Sterilization
Tying of the ovarian tubes in female dogs (tubal ligation) and of the spermatic cord in males (vasectomy) in order to prevent conception. Not to be confused with castration (qv) or spaying (qv).

Styptic
Medication to stop bleeding.

Sulfa drugs
Drugs that act similarly to antibiotics (qv), inhibiting the growth and multiplication of bacteria.

Thrombosis
The clogging of arteries or veins by blood clots, primarily in the coronary arteries (heart infarct).

Transfusion
Transfer of blood from one dog to another. The transfusion is made intravenously.

Tuberculin test
A skin test that shows whether the organism has antibodies against tuberculosis.

Ultrasound
Examination of internal organs using an ultrasound device that electronically processes reflected ultrasound waves into visual images. Other ultrasound devices are used to clean tartar off teeth and to disperse particles of liquids (aerosols) for inhalation therapy (qv).

Uremia
A state of self-poisoning by the body with urinary substances. Brought about by severe kidney disease or kidney failure.

Vaccination
Injection of vaccines that create immunity in the body through the production of antibodies (active vaccination) or injection of antisera that contain antibodies against certain diseases (passive vaccination).

X-ray pictures
Photographic images recorded on film (negative) as electromagnetic radiation (X-rays) briefly passes through parts of the body.

X-rays
High-energy, ionizing electromagnetic radiation capable of penetrating solids and thus suitable for giving a visual picture of body parts. If overused, they can cause radiation damage.

Zoonosis
A disease communicable from animals to humans, such as rabies and toxoplasmosis.

Index

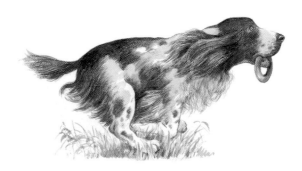

Information

Useful Books
For further reading on this subject and related matter, consult the following books also published by Barron's Educational Series, Inc.

Alderton, David: *The Dog Care Manual,* 1986.
Frye, Frederic: *First Aid for Your Dog,* 1987.
Klever, Ulrich: *The Complete Book of Dog Care,* 1989.

Animal Protection
American Society for the Prevention of Cruelty to Animals (ASPCA)
424 East 92 Street
New York, NY 10128
(212) 876-7700

Homeopathic Veterinary Referral
American Holistic Veterinary Medical Association
2214 Old Emmorton Road
Bel Air, MD 21015

Liability Insurance
Almost all insurance companies now offer liability insurance policies for dogs. Check with them about health insurance as well.

The Author
Dr. Uwe Streitferdt, specialist in veterinary science for small animals. He studied veterinary medicine and served for seven years as scientific assistant at the Medical and Surgical Animal Clinic of the University of Munich. Since 1978 he has had a practice for small animals in Munich. He is a consultant for magazines, radio, and television.

Contributing Authors
Christine Metzger has been working as a freelance journalist since 1985 and has many publications to her credit. Ms. Metzger wrote the following sections: A Healthy Dog, The Proper Diet, Practical Advice for Dog Owners, Preventive Care, Care of a Sick Dog, Getting Ready to See the Veterinarian, Behavioral Problems, Estrus and Birth.

Dr. Claus-Michael Pautzke, specialist in veterinary surgery and homeopathy, has been practicing homeopathic medicine for animals for 15 years. Dr. Pautzke wrote the section Homeopathy for Dogs and the suggestions for homeopathic treatment in the descriptions of the diseases.

Poisoning Information
In most large cities there are information centers you can call in case of poisoning. Although they are intended for people, you can also call them if your dog is poisoned. Obtain the Poison Control Center telephone number and keep it handy.

Photo Credits
Animal Photography/Wilbie: Page 61; Animal Photography/Thompson: Page 53; Bender: Page 17; Brozio: Pages 8, 105; Groger: Inside front cover, page 36; Gunzel: Front cover, page 128; Info Hund/Kramer: Page 40; IPO: Page 13, below; Junior/Fellner: Back cover; Junior/Liebold: Pages 9, 112; Junior/Speisen: Page 68; Layer: Page 80; Mahler: Pages 89, left and right, 90, 91, 100; Meier: Pages 65, 76, 108, left, middle, right, 109, above and below; Nicaise: Pages 37, left and right; 55, 69, 72, 73, 81, 84; Reinhard: Pages 45, 104, above and below; Schmidbauer: Page 13, above; Silverstris/Kerscher: Page 12; Silverstris/Lenz: Page 16; Silverstis/Wothe: Pages 93, 96/97.

Important Notes

This book is about treating dog diseases. The suggestions and methods of treatment are based on the authors' many years of practical experience. But since every case is different, not every suggestion can have unlimited validity. In spite of the detailed and comprehensive descriptions, the book lays no claim to completeness. That is why it is absolutely necessary to visit the veterinarian if there are complications.

Substances that contain insecticides (see Medicated Baths and Rubbing Medication into the Skin, page 23) have to be handled with great caution. Wearing rubber gloves is recommended, especially for persons with sensitive skin or a tendency to develop allergies.

Some diseases of dogs, namely, ringworm (page 81), rabies and leptospirosis (page 99), parasites (such as roundworms, page 101), and imported diseases, such as Leishmaniasis (page 102) can be transmitted to humans. Maintain hygienic conditions and, if you suspect a problem, visit your physician. Tell him or her that you have a dog and what disease the dog has.

© Copyright 1993 by Gräfe und Unzer GmbH, Munich.

The title of the German book is *Mein Kranker Hund.*

Translated from the German by Robert and Rita Kimber.

First English language edition published in 1994 by Barron's Educational Series, Inc.

English translation © Copyright 1994 by Barron's Educational Series, Inc.

Address all inquiries to:
Barron's Educational Series, Inc.
250 Wireless Boulevard
Hauppauge, New York 11788

Library of Congress Catalog Card No. 93-41249

International Standard Book Number 0-8120-1842-7

PRINTED IN HONG KONG

4567   9927   987654321

Library of Congress Cataloging-in-Publication Data

Streitferdt, Uwe.
    [Mein Kranker Hund. English]
    Healthy dog, happy dog : a complete guide to dog diseases and their treatment : first aid-treatment-care / Uwe Streitferdt; contributing authors, Christine Metzger, Claus-Michael Pautzke; drawings by Gyorgy Jankovics and color photos by renowned animal photographers.
        p.   cm.
    Includes bibliographical references (p.   ) and index.
    ISBN 0-8120-1842-7
    1. Dogs—Diseases. 2. Dogs—Diseases—Alternative treatment. 3. Dogs—Health. 4. Homeopathic veterinary medicine. I. Metzger, Christine. II. Pautzke, Claus-Michael. III. Title.
SF991.S87513   1994   93-41249
636.7'0896—dc20   CIP

First Aid for Dogs

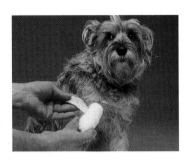

*A*ccidents happen suddenly. If your dog gets hurt, its fate depends on your ability to make the right decisions and act quickly. Your first rule should be to stay calm and act thoughtfully even though you feel like panicking at the sight of the injured dog. By taking some appropriate emergency measures you can prevent further damage or complications. After providing this first aid you will have to take the dog to the veterinarian as soon as possible.

Prolapse of the Eyeball

In short-nosed dogs fights sometimes result in the eye bulging out between the lids because the short skull hardly protects the eyes at all. Try to replace the eye by pulling the lids over the globe again. If you don't succeed, put a head bandage over the eye and transport the dog to the veterinarian immediately.

Head Bandage

If there are injuries to the eyeball or heavily bleeding wounds to the ears, an emergency head bandage may be necessary. Place a tissue on the wound and a bandage—preferably of gauze—around the head in a way to exert pressure on the injured place. Run the bandage around the other ear once in front and once in back. This way it won't slip out of place.

Foreign Body in the Mouth

When chewing on sticks and bones dogs can get splinters stuck between the molars (see also page 42). Take the dog to the veterinarian.

Cuts on the Paws

If the paw is bleeding badly you have to put on a pressure bandage. First clean the wound of dirt and foreign bodies. Then cover it with a compress (a piece of clean cloth or a tissue). Wrap the paw tightly with a bandage or a strip of cloth.